DON'T ASK ME HOW I'M DOING

Life, Death, and Everything in Between

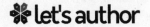

❄ let's author

"This book is a gift. A very generous gift, written beautifully by courageous, intelligent, expressive young people sharing their stories of dealing with cancer.

It covers themes that include the discovery stage, with all its shock, anger and grieving; to living with cancer while managing mental and physical health; to the challenges of parenting with cancer; and letting loved ones go.

We are immediately pulled into a world we are too afraid to ask about. Perhaps we just don't know what to say when we learn someone has cancer; perhaps it reminds us of our own mortality; perhaps we would just prefer not to think about things that are uncomfortable. Well, too bad. You cannot ignore this book and what it's trying to do. It's time to confront our own discomfort, to admit we don't know enough, and we need urgently to think about what is most important in our lives.

This book will resonate deeply with those living with cancer, and those who have lost loved ones to it. But really, it is for everyone: we can learn what it's like to be on the inside when someone's world is being rocked and turned upside down; to develop new compassion and presence, to listen more than we talk and to support in meaningful ways. And importantly, to ask ourselves about our own lives, accept our mortality and live more meaningfully. That is one heck of a gift."

— **Yashodhara Lal**,
Best-Selling Author of *How I Became a Farmer's Wife*,
Harper Collins, 2018

"Don't ask me how I am doing!

Firstly, what a title!

I find this book a compelling read once you have gone through the initial turmoil "to read or not to read"! This is not a book you will typically pick up and read by choice. It will have to be thrust upon you, either by fate, circumstance or by chance. Written evocatively by a whole lot of heroes who have braved the dreaded C word. Once you have gone through the stories of trysts, trials and tribulations, you emerge with a whole new mindset to cancer. And more importantly a positive and winning mindset "against", "to" and "of" cancer.

The fact remains. Life is always lived in denial. Denial of the fact that the end reality is death. To that extent, the key question is, are we living? Or are we dying, one day at a time? The answer is certainly blowing in the wind.

Life is really a scale. While some scales are longer, some are shorter. There is a clear beginning and a clear end. And the fact is that no one really knows whose scale is shorter and whose longer. And by how much.

What happens when the alarm-clock of mortality goes off all of a sudden? Do we get jolted, and how! And how do we really react? And do we then look at life and all its joys differently?

"Don't Ask Me How I'm Doing" is this classic book. An insider's view of a sudden mortality jolt. I do believe this is a must-read book for all. What happens to all the heroes (gender neutral) in this book can happen to any of us.

It's a good read. A read that possibly puts us in a place where we must belong. But don't."

— Harish Bijoor,
Business and Brand-Strategy Specialist

"This is the kind of book you may not want to read and yet when you do it's unputdownable. Apart from the novelty of the theme - of young adults fighting against, surviving and living with Cancer, it's brutally honest in articulation and brilliant in execution. Touching, poignant, humorous, optimistic, the book is a roller coaster much like the emotions of its protagonists. The authors, while being brutally frank about their experiences, hopes and fears, also show commendable temperament and maturity far beyond their ages, in describing their mental, physical and psychological struggles against the Big C. Each story is different but each author is in sparkling form. Together their stories are inspiring and give us much to hope, laugh and see life in a different light."

— Srikant Kesnur,
Director, Maritime Warfare Centre (MWC), Mumbai

First Printing: December 2022

Hardcover ISBN: 978-81-952590-5-2
Paperback ISBN: 978-81-952590-4-5
Ebook ISBN: 978-81-952590-6-9

Illustrations by Suman Kaur
All Illustrations are for representational purpose only.
Cover Design by Manoj Vijayan
Typeset by Manoj Gupta
Edited by Ananya Bhatia

LetsAuthor
www.letsauthor.com

TABLE OF CONTENTS

Navigating College and Career

Exploring Existential Questions

Finances, Insurance, and Hospitals

Following Caregivers' Journeys

When a Caregiver Gets Cancer

INTRODUCTION

I landed in Boston on August 29, 2021, unpacked my stuff in the dorm, and decided to hang out with some newly made friends. We were dancing in their newly rented house to celebrate our arrival at Harvard. While we were at it, suddenly, I froze and fell down, hitting my head hard. The next thing I remember is being dragged to the bathroom. Blink one. I've locked myself in. Blink two. I'm inside an ambulance. Blink three. I'm being wheeled into an emergency room.

The next 48 hours are a blur. I have vague memories of several beeping machines, IV injections, blood tests, and a CT scan. In a brief spell of consciousness, the nurses informed me that a violent seizure had landed me in the ER and they had found "something" in my brain. After what felt like forever, the same ambulance took me to another hospital to get an MRI scan.

Post MRI, a young doctor solemnly told me that they had found a glioma. Confused, I asked him to explain.

"You have a brain tumor that needs to be removed immediately. It seems cancerous. If it is, you may not survive for more than five years. I'm really sorry," he said.

"But my master's program at Harvard starts tomorrow," I said softly.

Tears had begun to trickle down my cheeks. I called up my brother-in-law and sister who live in Atlanta, muttering something incoherent at first. Finally, uttering the "C word" out loud for the first time, I asked my sister to inform our parents. I didn't have the strength to wipe the smile off their faces. Thousands of miles away, I can only wonder how shocked and helpless they must have felt. When the neurosurgeon arrived to prep me for emergency surgery, I told him that my parents were doctors and I wished to be treated in India. After my father spoke to him, he reluctantly discharged me. The decision to move back—putting my decade-long dream on hold in the hope of surviving and being well enough to return someday—was gut-wrenching.

As soon as I landed after my 30-hour-long flight, I hugged my parents tight and all of us teared up. Over the next couple of weeks, we met many, many doctors and after several discussions, I was finally scheduled for a craniotomy—an extremely dangerous surgery where they drill into and cut open the skull to operate on the brain. When I was wheeled out of the operating room after a 7-hour-long surgery, they had successfully removed the whole tumor. My post-op recovery was great and, 72 hours later, I was sent home. Things were beginning to look up.

A fortnight later, in a weird twist of fate, my biopsy reports informed us that my tumor was caused by a rare type of chronic brain cancer. We sincerely hoped it would be benign. It was devastating news. However, there was one silver lining—it grew slowly and I had all the favorable genetic and molecular markers that make it responsive to treatment every time it recurs. I cried tears of joy. At least I had more time than I had been informed. Five years had seemed like nothing at all. The next couple of months were spent recuperating at home.

However, life after was far more difficult than I imagined. There was no roadmap available. Indian cancer support groups, both the general ones and the ones exclusively for brain cancers, often didn't have enough people of my age or resources for the challenges I was facing—navigating life with cancer as a young person. Some resources were available online, but they were from the West and none of them were completely relatable or answered my questions adequately.

There is a huge gap in the Indian and South Asian cancer ecosystem—almost no attention is given to young adults who are in a period of life when one hits several developmental milestones such as finishing school and college, starting and growing at work, making friends and creating networks, forming relationships and getting married, having and raising children, etc.

Exactly a month before my 30th birthday, I stumbled upon a post by the open authoring platform through which this book is being published. They were looking for non-traditional writers and I pitched an idea about co-authoring a book on the lived experiences of young Indian folks between ages of 17 and 39 on "adulting with cancer" since several of our challenges cut across different types, stages, grades, and treatment regimens. That's the origin story of this book.

In an age of toxic positivity and inspiration porn that expects trauma survivors to carry the burden of being the heroes of their own journeys, this book aims to paint a much more real, raw, honest yet hopeful take on what it actually feels and looks like to be a young adult cancer patient, survivor, and caregiver.

I thank all the co-authors for generously sharing their vulnerable selves, warts and all, in a quest to help those who desperately want to hear stories of how others like them dealt with these common challenges in their own unique ways and continue to do so. We hope, through our stories, you will realize you're not alone, not weird, and not insufficient for struggling to figure out how to get back to life or establish your "new normal." It's a tough journey with many potholes and speed breakers that may or may not lead to thriving or becoming the next role model. We continue to play with the cards we've been dealt in life, no matter the odds. Even if you are in no way related to cancer, we hope our stories give you a peek into how becoming aware of your mortality changes you as a person forever.

People have asked me what the title of the book means. We in the young adult cancer community are often asked "How are you doing?", not because someone really wants to know but as a form of politically correct small talk or conversation starter similar to "Hey! What's up?". Many don't really want to know what's *truly* going on. If we dare to actually respond honestly and say that we're going through a rough patch or are having a bad day, we're met with shock, awkward silence, or offered unwarranted advice. How most people instead expect us to respond is some version of "I'm good. How are you?" Very few genuinely care to *listen* to what we have to say and make time for it. Tired of this fake pleasantry, I decided to name this book *Don't Ask Me How I'm Doing*. The subtitle, "Life, Death, and Everything in Between," encapsulates the breadth of our experiences. This doesn't mean the next time you meet someone who has or had cancer, you can't ask them the question. However, do it only if you really mean it—ask this question only when you honestly want to know how they are and have the time to listen, without interrupting or jumping to offer advice. Else, use other neutral conversation starters like "Hey! What's up?"

Life is a journey towards death. As they say, the goal isn't to reach the destination but to enjoy the process. Everyone has an expiry date. Compared to others, I'm just more aware of how close mine probably is. Hence, I live life with an urgency that I am on borrowed time, unsure what tomorrow brings or how long I'll live. I had told myself that if I survived the surgery, I would live a more meaningful life. Leading the effort to get this book written and published is my attempt to make a tiny difference in the lives of Indian and South Asian young adults who deal with cancer.

—Sanjay Deshpande

SOCIAL AND RELATIONSHIP ISSUES

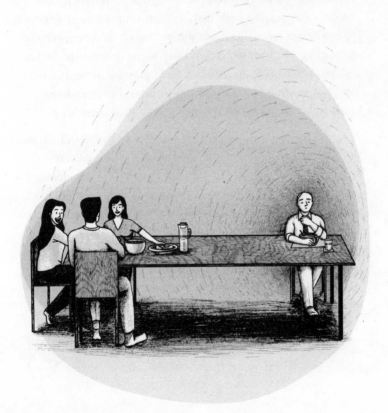

Many in the young adult cancer community believe "What doesn't kill you, makes you weirder and harder to relate to." This is because rarely any experience compares to what you go through when you have or had cancer. Often it is terribly isolating due to the toxic feeling of constantly being misunderstood. Your parents, siblings, partner, and friends, no one can truly comprehend what you are struggling with. Not to forget the taboo associated with it that often results in a gag order from your own families. You might lose or distance yourself from some old friends, grow closer to those who you never thought you would, and make a few new ones along the way. You start valuing your near and dear ones who truly make an effort to be there for you through the good and bad days.

Cancer makes it awkward to socialize and maintain relationships. Most people don't know what to say to us and in an attempt to be politically correct, they either avoid addressing the elephant in the room or ghost you till they can figure out what to say, which may take months, years or probably forever. In fact, talking about "it" can make people queasy. It might remind some of the fragility of life, their own mortality or burst their bubble of invincibility. Here are a few stories about how some of the co-authors navigated these turbulent waters and other related challenges in their own ways.

COMING OUT OF THE CANCER CLOSET

I'm not into hiding stuff. If you ever look into my closet, apart from my perfectly ironed clothes, neatly folded and stacked up according to type, you will find my prized collection of printed boxers and underpants proudly displayed instead of being tucked away in some corner. Some call it being bold but I always wear my "secrets" on my sleeve; if you know, you know what I mean. But here's the paradox: I'm also extremely anxious. It's a huge conundrum—choosing to live my truth or worrying about its consequences; my version of "to be or not to be." I often find myself in the middle, being pulled in one direction or the other. However, over the years, I have realized that being vulnerable takes far more courage than projecting strength. So here I am, spilling the beans or tea, based on whatever your age might be.

The Quintessential Question: Why Me?

When I was first informed that I could have cancer, my immediate reaction was to think I was being pranked. In my defense, I had watched way too many episodes of *Just for Laughs Gags* where unassuming people in the West were pranked and their reactions were filmed. But when the doctor didn't laugh or point to any secret cameras, it quickly dawned on me that this wasn't staged. Like a deer caught in headlights, I found myself utterly shocked and frozen in fear.

Here I was, a healthy 29-year-old, freshly landed in the US to live the "American Dream," who suddenly, out of nowhere, found out that he possibly had brain cancer. As I lay in the ER contemplating life and death, instead of looking forward to my year at Harvard, I was going through a monumental crisis. In retrospect, it makes for a great story with natural plot twists. Maybe I'll write that memoir someday and someone will eventually turn it into a movie! Perhaps my childhood dream of being famous will finally come true. Jokes apart, one question has gnawed at me for a long time, "Why me?"

I thought my doctors would have some answers but they didn't. Assuming they were just trying to keep me in the dark so that I didn't blame myself, I took to the internet. There are only three known risk factors. Some are hereditary whereas a few others are caused by rare genetic disorders. But no one in my family had brain cancer, nor did they or I have any genetic disorder. The only other known cause was exposure to high levels of ionizing radiation. I don't think getting one CT scan as a child when I hit my head in school counts as hazardous. I even tried finding out if any of my relatives had cancer. After vigorously shaking the family tree, I found two on each side—on my father's side, someone in their 70s had the stomach type and another in their 40s had the blood type; on my mother's side, someone had the lung kind in their 60s and another had the stomach kind in their 70s. It was a pointless exercise; the apple had fallen far away from the tree. Clearly, none of their illnesses were related to mine.

When the doctors and the internet failed me, my parents joined the bandwagon of unearthing the answer to my question. We wondered if my cancer could be the result of poisonous levels of air pollution in the cities I had lived in during the last decade—Mumbai for four years and Delhi for seven years. Choosing to live in these cities was akin to willfully inflicting self-harm; I had done so for the sake of my education and career. Professionally, I reaped dividends but the success came at a huge personal cost. While I can't say that this was the exact reason for my ill health, I know it certainly didn't help.

Now that my parents too couldn't find an answer to my elusive question, my grandmother chimed in, "It must be the toxic pesticides used to grow produce these days, probably why the organic food industry thrives promising fruits and vegetables grown without pesticides." Unconvinced that these answers held any ground, I approached my therapist. Her theory was that it could be because of my childhood trauma. Looking back, I didn't think being molested by an older man and bullied by my peers could cause physical diseases, especially the "Big C." I had only assumed that such traumatic experiences would have led me to suffer from severe mental health issues that I now have—low stress tolerance, constant vigilance, and high-functioning anxiety. But never did I think that poor mental health could cause cancer. Although recent evidence shows a strong correlation between the two, there is no evidence that the former causes the latter. However, I convinced myself that it might have played a small part.

When all these answers or reasons pointed in no particular direction, I started blaming my lifestyle. General medical advice suggests that poor dietary choices, lack of exercise, irregular sleeping patterns, and consumption of alcohol and tobacco compounds the risk of developing cancer. Basically, everything a young 20-something does to have fun. But I didn't do anything different from my peers. So, why did I get it and not any of them? Did I do something significantly worse? There weren't any answers, no matter how hard I looked.

As soon as I exhausted all the logical reasons I could think of, I took to whimsical thinking. Maybe it was divine payback for not praying for a decade? Maybe I was cursed for having lived with two black cats that my previous flatmate had? Maybe someone had given me the evil eye, jealous of my success? Perhaps it was just bad karma—maybe I was being punished for doing some horrible things in the past or in my previous lives?

Obviously, I was aware of how irrational these thoughts were. However, I couldn't help but wonder, could there be any truth to them? When faced with mortality, you tend to look beyond reason and reality and consider the possibility that humans and science may not have all the answers. I briefly turned to faith to find some but realized maybe it was just fate. Life's a gamble and I had landed up with bad luck. For an anxious person, nothing's scarier than ambiguity, uncertainty, and lack of control. Unfortunately, all three were simultaneously in action here—literally my worst nightmare.

I haven't made peace with not knowing why I ended up getting cancer and keep Googling for answers on days I'm down in the dumps, but I have reluctantly, more or less, accepted that I may never really know. I like to believe that each of us is a thread in the large tapestry that makes up human history—some long, others short, all necessary nonetheless. Arriving at this conclusion is my "coming of age" story—a journey from invincibility to humility.

What Skeletons Are You Hiding in Your Closet?

Once I was finally diagnosed, I went through a rollercoaster of emotions. All my life, I had been waiting for the other shoe to drop. I knew something was coming but didn't know what. I was constantly vigilant, looking over my shoulder, double checking any symptoms that seemed out of the ordinary, and being extra careful while I did everything. In a way, I had been preparing for some catastrophe all my life and it had finally occurred. It took me a while to get over the shock. But as someone who prepares for the worst and hopes for the best, I accepted the situation, armed myself with all the information I could find on what to expect, and researched the best course of treatment that currently existed for people like me.

No one wants their child to suffer such a fate. Even though they were doctors themselves, it took my parents quite a while to adapt to this new reality. My father is not very talkative. While I did talk to him often about the latest medical research and new prognosis statistics, I couldn't really figure out what was going on in his head. He was worried and it showed on his otherwise poker face. Yet, he was able to make peace with the situation quicker, I think, than my more outspoken and animated mother. She knew what a malignant tumor meant but was in denial about the fact that there was no cure; she kept insisting that since I was done with my treatment and was tumor-free, I should move on with my life. She wasn't willing to entertain the thought that it could recur, require more aggressive treatment, and leave more deficits in its wake. I tried putting myself in her shoes. It was beyond heartbreaking to even imagine what she was going through. So, I decided to give her time and space to come around. She eventually did.

"Don't tell anyone you have cancer. EVER," she issued a gag order right after. I was confused because she knew that I had a non-communicable disease that I had played no part in getting. So far, the only people who knew were my parents, my sister, her husband, and my best friends. I was asked not to inform others, especially anyone in my extended family. But I really wanted to tell my grand-mother that my tumor was not benign as the world thought it to be. I couldn't hold back my tears every time she said, "Close this chapter and move forward."

I had to fight with my mother to be allowed to tell my grand-mother and a few close cousins. I argued that with a potentially shorter lifespan, I wanted to finally live life on my own terms with-out constantly adjusting or filtering myself due to the fear of "*log kya kahenge*" (what will people think). I either managed to convince her or just guilt-tripped her; either way, she let me go ahead.

When I finally revealed the news, most of my relatives were shell-shocked. "Don't say it out loud and don't think about the fact that you have it. Just think you are well and you will be," they said. While I knew they meant well, it felt like my illness and suffering were being dismissed. I tried to explain why what they said didn't help me and found out that they only had two replies—"Don't admit it and it'll go away" or "You'll be okay because you are so young." They literally didn't have the vocabulary to respond in any other way.

Cancer, like many other life-threatening illnesses, shatters the veneer of our invincibility and reveals the fragility of life. It reminds us that we are mortal beings who will die one day. But we as a society don't like talking about death, especially not our own or that of our loved ones. It makes us uneasy because we believe talking about it would somehow hasten it. While some equate cancer with dying, thanks to the advances in medicine, many different types of cancer are now curable or at least have treatments that significantly extend lifespan and improve the quality of life. Recent research suggests that the kind I have might become completely curable in the next decade or so. Nothing wrong in hoping for a miracle, right?

When the rest of my relatives found out that I had abruptly moved back to India from the US, they inquired with my parents. The answer remained the same, even after the biopsy report had confirmed that my tumor was malignant—"He had a brain tumor which has been removed, and now he's okay." At home, I tried to confront the huge elephant in the room: they implied that my tumor was benign and I was fine. I understood the need to keep family matters private, but I didn't understand why they felt a sense of shame and anxiety in admitting the truth.

It's 2022 and the C-word is still a huge taboo, even in educated Indian families. Some people falsely believe it is contagious and can spread. Others inaccurately think that if someone has any form of malignancy, others in their family could also get it, so people want to stay away—not wanting to marry anyone remotely related. It is also considered an old person's disease, like heart attacks, brain strokes, Parkinson's, and Alzheimer's. So, when a young person gets it, the stigma magnifies. This fear pressurizes the patient to keep it a secret, lest the rest of their family suffers as a result. This explains my family's fear of being discriminated against and ostracized, if anyone found out the truth.

Publicly Coming Out of the Cancer Closet

I've always been a bit of a firebrand rebel, much to my parents' dismay. In the past, I have acted boldly in the face of adversity.

Never did I silently accept any form of injustice, even if it didn't affect me. I've always challenged outdated social norms and stood up for my values. Obviously, I wasn't going to keep my diagnosis a secret. Making my family and myself suffer in silence and isolation wouldn't really help anyone. I wanted to speak openly about it, raise awareness that this could happen to anyone, and do something to serve the community to which I now belonged.

When my mother realized she wouldn't be able to stop me, she practically begged me to at least wait a while before I told the extended family. I relented. All my friends knew by then anyway. But three months after the surgery, when my first post-op MRI scan came clean, I was ready to re-enter the land of the well, leaving the land of the ill behind. It was then that I decided to put up a LinkedIn post narrating my ordeal, disclosing my status, and asking for leads for part-time/consulting work. I was fully aware that once I did this, there was no going back. In the world of the internet, information once revealed can never be erased. Thousands of people would read and share the post, making it public knowledge in some form and shape for eternity.

I briefly contemplated the effect this would have on my career and my personal life—I probably wouldn't be able to hide it from my future employers who might be biased, severely affecting the kind of job opportunities I could get. I wouldn't even be able to prevent someone from finding out, even if I didn't want them to know, in case they decided to look me up online. But I wanted to break the taboo and normalize talking about a life-threatening disease such as cancer publicly. Thankfully, I had prior experience in talking publicly about issues that personally affected me. In hindsight, talking about the disease reduced the pool of opportunities, but it also helped me filter out the ones that were definitely not a good cultural fit and didn't align with my values. Eventually, this decision helped me find better workplaces. There's a caveat though. I had a safety net that prevented me from worrying about not finding work: I had enough professional credibility through the skills, experience, and connections I had built throughout my career so far. As an alum of two of India's best colleges, St. Xavier's College, Mumbai, and Ashoka University, Delhi NCR, and having a deferred admission from the world's best higher education institution, Harvard University, I had access to strong networks. Fully aware of my privilege, I wanted to put it to good use.

In my head, the math was clear. The benefits outweighed the risks, no matter the outcome. So, I went ahead and put up a post. Instead of becoming a source of discrimination, the post went viral. Many reshared it, offering to connect me with the right people and helping me get several leads. After speaking to a few, I joined an organization that met my needs, aligned with my values, and offered me the necessary flexibility. I worked for a couple of months and realized that I was not being treated differently. However, it also dawned on me that I needed to reset the priorities in my life. While I was doing work that pre-cancer Sanjay would have truly enjoyed, the post-cancer Sanjay didn't find it as meaningful. I had to recalibrate my thoughts regarding what I wanted to do with my life. I'll talk more about this in another chapter.

I decided to take the next leap of faith. On the six-month anniversary of my diagnosis, I put up a post on Facebook and Instagram narrating my experience. Once it was out there, it felt like a huge weight had been lifted off my chest. I no longer had to pretend everything was A-okay, and I was able to raise awareness that even someone as young and healthy as me could get it. However, it was an awkward balancing act. I was out of the cancer closet to the rest of the world but was still hiding it from my own extended family who weren't connected with me on any of the social media platforms.

My parents were also in the dark about everything that I had been up to. When I finally told them I had decided to write this book, they were thrilled that I wanted to be a published writer but not so much about revealing my diagnosis to the whole world. As the website page for the book went live and the tentative book cover was designed, things started to change. I told a few cousins that I was working on a book. They were excited and wanted to know what I was writing about. I explained the vision of the book and shared the website link. All of them were supportive and appreciated my initiative. They reached out to my parents and told them how proud they were of what I was doing. This changed things for my parents. They voluntarily started telling our relatives that I was writing a book, even showing off the book cover and sharing the website link. They were surprised to see the amount of love and support my effort was garnering. Instead of feeling shame and hiding my illness, they were embracing the fact that I was channeling my energy to positively make a difference in the lives of others like me.

This was the tipping point. I no longer cared who knew or didn't, who thought or said what about me. I was now completely out of the cancer closet, with the unwavering support of my family.

Coming out is never a one-time event. You have to keep revealing your status to new people for the rest of your life if you think they matter or need to know. There's also no telling how they'll respond. I hate having to repeat myself, at least to the ones I know or who know me, which is why I prefer being publicly out. Hence, my decision to reveal my status to everyone on social media and through this book. I also got a beautiful, difficult-to-ignore tattoo on my right forearm on my 30th birthday to commemorate my experience. It's a top view of the brain's hemispheres with flowers growing out of the right side where my tumor was excavated from with the text "seize the day" under it, a pun on my seizures and a mantra for life—do all that you want to do now because the future isn't promised. Pretty in-your-face, I've been told. However, I have several cancer buddies in my age group who don't choose to be "out" like me. My ability to do so is based on several intersectional privileges I enjoy, which I am aware of and acknowledge openly. Others prefer to keep their status to a close circle of family and friends and maybe their immediate team at work. Some even choose not to reveal it at all, especially if they have been cured. A few worry that letting people know might adversely affect their career and romantic lives, which might be a fair assessment.

Using the relevant vocabulary while coming out is another delicate yet significant decision you make after much deliberation. People with cancer choose to use different labels to identify themselves and communicate their status. Some call themselves "patients" even after active treatment because, well, if you are not cured completely, you are still a patient. But this makes me feel perennially sick. Others call themselves "fighters/warriors," suggesting they are battling an enemy. However, the malignant cells are not an external threat, they are a part of your own body, so how can I say that I am at war with myself? A few call themselves "thrivers," indicating that they are prospering or flourishing due to or in spite of their cancer. This puts too much pressure to perform feats for the world to feel inspired. I steer clear of this one completely. Then there's "terminal," which means someone has tried everything and is at the end of their life. Again, not true for me. Most call themselves "survivors," suggesting that they live on despite coming close to death, and it is the most commonly used term for all those who are done with treatment, even if they aren't completely cured. This somewhat resonates with me—brain cancer survivor. Lastly, there's "living with chronic cancer," indicating that their type is similar to chronic illness like type 2 diabetes that requires following precautions and needs active treatment only when it flares up once in a while. This comes closest to my reality since chances are that my type might rear its ugly head sometime in the future but can be treated if it does. Based on my current health status I've created "living well with chronic cancer." I use the last two interchangeably as appropriate—brain cancer survivor or living well with chronic cancer.

The Unvarnished Truth

I have simplified my journey for the sake of brevity. It certainly wasn't this linear and was punctuated with several bouts of grief and depression. I want to paint an honest picture and not shy away from admitting that it hurt like hell at times and I was often a mess. A pendulum would be an accurate representation of my actual journey, swinging between the good days and the bad days. Do I ever regret telling the world? Sometimes, especially when I consider my career and dating prospects, one of which I will cover in more detail in another chapter.

I also worry if I have in some ways made my diagnosis my identity/identifier—I'm the man who has/had brain cancer. But very few experiences in life affect you this way. So, I tell myself that while I have multiple identities, this just happens to be the most salient one that affects every aspect of my life for the rest of it, hence, it's okay. There is no single way to deal with whether you choose to disclose your diagnosis, including to whom, when, how, and where. I hope my story illustrates one way to do so and helps you figure out if this works for you.

—Sanjay Deshpande

DANCING WITH MY TRIBE

Sometimes the most powerful voice is the most silent. And, the biggest support is the quiet unwavering kind. The support that does not need words and rises above the chatter in your head. The "no matter what" support. This is my ode to a few beautiful souls. Those who have lit the way for me through the darkness like fireflies and never let me feel alone.

Best Friend 1: How are you doing? Call me.

Dad: Beta, what did the doctor say? How are you feeling now?

Friend 2: Hi Snehal, I just got to know from Mahima what happened. I don't know what to say. Are you okay?

Waiting to meet my doctor, I sighed as I scrolled through the messages. My mind was screaming, *Leave me alone! What kind of a question is 'how are you doing?' I have cancer, goddammit. Would I be celebrating?*

It had been two months. I was tired of this incessant barrage of messages and missed calls I had been receiving since my diagnosis.

Why can't people get the hint, I am ghosting them. Because I don't want to talk to them or to anybody! I don't need their sympathy or their self-proclaimed medical analysis of my situation that I will get well soon!

For the umpteenth time, I thanked God that I wasn't in India. I could avoid the melodrama that would have followed this news. I could literally see people do a triple take, like in Indian soaps, "Kya!

Kya! Kya!" (What! What! What!), frequently used to demonstrate shock.

I wiped away the stray tear which seemed to roll down so often those days. Only 5% of women who get breast cancer are below the age of 40, and here I was, in the fellowship of the chosen few. This gift was bestowed on me at 37, when we had just shifted from India to Singapore and my baby was 4 months old.

The first month after the diagnosis was just a series of activities—finding the right doctor, taking multiple opinions, and getting a number of tests, needle pricks, and more done. But with Stage 4 cancer, with the disease spreading to my lungs, liver, and bone, time was not a luxury I had.

Now with the treatment in full swing, I was nervously beginning this new way of life. I was in shock. And then, to be asked, "How did it happen?", "How are you feeling?", "Are you doing okay?"—questions to which I did not have any answers—was discomforting, to say the least.

It was difficult to even look at people and not feel pangs of anger and envy.

What do you know about pain and facing death in the face? I would silently ask people this question as I walked past them.

I felt abnormal; I felt as if everyone, but me, seemed to have it easy. I was surrounded by a whirlwind of these thoughts, I had no one who I thought would understand me. No one I could turn to, who would just say, "I get it!"

I could see my inner child sitting in a corner, hugging her knees, and weeping. I wanted nothing more than to be left alone. At the same time, I felt lonely, isolated, and targeted.

"Hi Snehal, how are you?" the doctor asked.

You really want to know doc? I laughed in my head.

"Snehal, you should join Breast Cancer Foundation, Singapore (BCF). You will meet other women there who are on a similar journey and I'm sure the foundation will be a great support system for you."

I almost blurted out, *I don't need more people in my life, I need a cure!*

But as I walked out of the clinic, I wrote to the BCF. Thus began my journey with a foundation that became one of my first support circles.

The first thing they did was put me in touch with a Befriender. Someone who had gone through a similar situation and who would journey with me for three months.

Befriender: Hi, Snehal. I understand what you are going through, and I hope I can be there for you in the way you would want me to. Let's talk when you are free.

With this simple message started a wonderful journey with someone whom I could relate to, talk to about my worries, ask all my silly questions, and just feel normal around. Every time we spoke, I would just be in awe of how calm she sounded. What a noble thing she was doing by putting herself out there to help others. All I wanted to do was hide away in my corner and never step out. Never let anyone know what was happening with me.

Within a few weeks of talking, she asked me if I would be comfortable joining the WhatsApp group for women with breast cancer below 40. She must have sensed my hesitation because she said,

"It's all right Snehal. You can take your time, but I am sure it will help you. Aren't you curious to meet others like us?"

I finally mumbled a yes and suddenly found myself amidst a flurry of online activity. As I introduced myself, I saw chats on cycling, queries on herbs, doctors, healing modalities, and so much more.

I was expecting a morbid group of women talking about mortality. Instead, I became a part of a vibrant tribe of wonderful and caring women.

Woman 1: Hey girl, welcome to the group. I too have a similar...

Woman 2: Hi Snehal. Let me know if you need anything.

Wait a minute, they seem so normal. Am I crazy to think I am abnormal? I'm not alone!

For the first time in almost two months, I no longer felt crazy and lonely. Some of these women were survivors, others were going through treatment, and some had been just diagnosed like me. Yet, it almost seemed as if they had a life beyond cancer; cancer was not their life.

The thing is, we all want to feel a part of a community. Sometimes we open up or find our space in the most unexpected of places. I felt I belonged here. Cancer was plaguing me with so many insecurities that seeing others like me leading seemingly regular lives was quite an eye opener.

They became my go-to source for all questions and worries. At other times, they were a source of inspiration. For the first time since my diagnosis, I learned to breathe easy and as I walked past strangers I would think, *Hmmm ... Maybe they all have a story I'm not aware of.*

I Needed Help! I Just Did Not Know It

Suruchi: Can we talk?

Me: No.

Suruchi: I just want to see how you are doing?

Me: I don't need help, Suruchi. I am fine.

Suruchi: You are doing the same thing you did during your divorce. Pushing me away because you think I live in some sort of a bubble. No one's life is perfect, Snehal. So don't assume it! You better get on the phone and speak with me!

Sigh. How is this girl able to get under my skin every time? I think that's what makes her a good counselor.

Grudgingly I called her the next day, and then the next week. Before I knew it, we were speaking regularly. I honestly don't remember when our casual chats seamlessly turned into beautiful therapeutic sessions.

I remember a particularly intense discussion with Suruchi. It was hard-hitting but at the same time it gave me a huge reality check.

"Who are you trying to get better for Snehal?" she inquired quietly.

"For my son, Samar, for my husband, and for my family," I said.

"I am just going to put something out there for you to think about. You don't need to respond to it," she said.

Oh God! Here come some pearls of wisdom, which I will have no clue what to do with. I am more of a diamond person.

"You need to get better for yourself! So that you can do everything you wish for with your loved ones," she said, stressing on the "you."

"You need to get better, not for others. But for you! How important is it for you to want to be here, happy and healthy, with them?" she continued.

So, this is what it feels like to have a "Kya! Kya! Kya!" moment! Now, how the hell am I supposed to process something like this, lady? Oh, but the lady wants to say more!

I could literally see her transforming into Master Oogway from *Kung Fu Panda*, carrying on with the sermon with her eyes closed, while I looked on as Po, the panda.

"Snehal, no one is obliged to do anything for you. Everyone is here for you because they want to be here. They want to see you well. Not out of sympathy, but empathy and because they love you."

Yes, master!

It dawned on me then that I had been so preoccupied worrying for my family that I had forgotten myself in the bargain. We speak so much about mental health every day, and yet often, forget our own mental well-being when it is most required.

This is when I slowly started looking for ways to take care of myself. The first thing I started doing was yoga, which I realized was doable through my treatment. Then I focused on my food. While the doctor did not recommend any particular diet for me, I decided to be more conscious about eating healthy.

I was also coping with severe body image issues. I hated how I looked post treatment and would avoid looking at myself in the mirror. But as days passed, I started realizing how much my body was coping with just to make me better. As part of my self-care routine, Suruchi made me write a letter to my body, as if it was a friend, appreciating it for what it added to my life and apologizing to it for everything I had and was putting it through. It was an extremely emotionally charged time for me, but it evoked such a new found appreciation for the way I felt about myself and my body.

She was helping me move slowly from my victim mode to taking charge. With each action, I felt like I was doing whatever was in my power to improve the situation. With each conversation, I started opening up to her more. It made me realize just how much I was in need of help. I was just too vain or ignorant to ask for it.

I was learning to reach out and be comfortable with it. As I extended my hand out more, I was grateful to see so many hands outstretched. This was when I started noticing how my family and friends had been silently supporting me.

My Inner Circle

Best Friend 1: Snehal! If you don't call me back, I am going to come to Singapore. May God help you then!

Dad: Dingu, call me. I am worried about you. I have not seen Samar, too, for quite some time.

Now my mind often behaves like Dr Jekyll and Mr Hyde, constantly in a dialogue.

Same pattern repeating, isn't it? Always shutting the door on your loved ones when you are in emotional turmoil. Why are you being so difficult? Why are you taking their support for granted?

Oh, all right, quit the lecture.

Me: Hi bestie. Sorry for not buzzing you... but can we just have a normal conversation? Like how we used to earlier? Tell me the latest gossip.

"Hi Dad... ," I called.

I blinked back tears, as I ended my call with Dad. It was hard not being in India, close to these people. It had barely been a year since we had moved to Singapore but so much had happened in this period that I never got the time to settle down.

Knock knock.

"Yes mom?" I hollered at my mother-in-law.

"I am taking Samar down to play. Do you need anything from the supermarket?" she asked.

My mom-in-law had come to stay with us before Samar was born. She was still here helping us raise him, while my husband and I focused on my treatment.

I was becoming aware of how my family and friends were working, almost invisibly, to make my life easier and to keep me happy.

So far, I guess, I had not been ready to see them, because of how sorry I felt for myself. And even though I pushed them away constantly, they had been relentless—my husband, my family, and my close friends.

My friends would set up Zoom meets with me during every chemo cycle, where we would gossip, laugh, and go crazy. They knew what I wanted and learned to be more patient with me.

My husband was like my knight in shining armor. He would accompany me for all my doctor visits, ensure that my random food cravings were satisfied, and just be there for me when my chips were down.

But as months passed, there seemed to be no respite. My treatment labored on and so did the cancer.

I remember once going to the clinic to get an update on my PET Scan. It had been eight months since my treatment had started, and I had already been through different chemotherapy drugs and hormonal treatments.

"Hi Sneeehal," the nurse greeted me as I waited. I was used to random pronunciations of my name, but I was sure she had added another "e" just for kicks.

"How have you been!" she asked, as she scanned her notes.

"I'm fine," I mumbled.

If every treatment change could be a new season, you could almost put Keeping Up with the Kardashians to shame, Sneeehal!' I smirked to myself. My mind usually went crazy after every scan. We had started calling it "Scanxiety." Usually, there is hope that things are getting better, but this time I was aware that we were just trying to understand how bad the spread was.

Sigh. The problems of metastatic breast cancer. The first time I had seen my scan, I was mesmerized by the number of lights it showed up. After that, I just prayed fervently for those lights to dim out. I think my body could definitely do with some darkness.

As my husband and I left the clinic, I felt myself tearing up. It was bad news again.

"When will this end? When can I just go back to normal? I can't deal with this anymore. I don't want to do this anymore. It's not fair." I was crying hysterically.

"This is not you, Snehal. You seem to have gone into hibernation, just playing a waiting game. Do something with your life. How long will you keep waiting?" he gently nudged.

Aah, I was wondering where you were, Master Shifu! Meet me, Po!

While I did not answer his question, I knew deep down that he was right. Honestly, I was tired of just waiting and not knowing. I just wanted to come unstuck.

When the Supported Became the Supporter

Me: I don't know if I can do it. It's too much for me.

Peer Coach 1: *Arey, main hoon na* (I am there for you). We will do it together. We'll earn our coaching certification together.

Peer Coach 2: Hey, I just found this great article on what we discussed last. I'm sure it will help!

I rolled my eyes as I thought, *Look, mom, I'm enjoying studying and complaining and doing homework! Hahaha.*

Post my husband's little talk, I had decided to pursue coaching that I had taken up as a part of my HR profession earlier.

I met a wonderful mentor, who despite my chemotherapy sessions, helped me complete my certification (almost 100 hours of training and practice). I met some wonderful peers who worked with me throughout the journey.

I met some amazing clients who made me feel that I could contribute to people's lives in a positive way. I was so grateful, that they trusted me with their vulnerabilities and dreams.

My family, as usual, stood rock solid behind me through this program. They knew it was rigorous and helped with Samar in every way possible.

With each passing day, I got more confident. I loved working with people through their challenges. Partnering with them in their journeys, just as I had been supported in mine.

I wanted to do more, touch more lives. Soon enough, BCF had an opportunity for me to share my story at a women's forum. I remember being so nervous, but I also knew it was my way of giving back. It took me back to how much I had appreciated my Befriender's help in those first few months. Maybe I could do it too.

I started sharing my story at various forums to spread breast cancer awareness. Many people started reaching out and sharing their personal stories, seeking help in areas they were struggling with or simply speaking their truth.

I had finally found a space to call my own. Slowly my life was changing. The supported was now becoming the supporter!

As I close this chapter, I don't have any pearls of wisdom to share. I just have stories and experiences. Stories of real people around me—my family, friends, BCF, and coaches who have been there for me through my cancer journey. All I had to do was make a little space for them in my life and allow them to co-exist with my thoughts.

Honestly, all of us have learned a lot in this journey. They learned to understand my needs better, and I learned to accept their love better. But most importantly, I just learned to smile.

—Snehal Ponde

THE IMPORTANCE OF FAMILY, GURU, AND FRIENDS IN CANCER

Gurur Brahma Gurur Vishnu Gurur Deva Maheshwara
Gurur Sakshat Param Brahma Tasmaye Sri Gurave Namah

[Guru (Teacher, Mentor, Guide) is akin to Brahma (The Creator),
Vishnu (The Preserver), and Maheshwara or Shiva (The Destroyer);

Guru is the embodiment *of Param Brahma* (the Limitless
all-encompassing cosmos) and I bow before thee Guru]

—Ancient Sanskrit sloka

In the family, he (the male head) *is the bourgeoisie* (the oppressor),
the woman represents the proletariat (oppressed).

—Friedrich Engels

Hi, a boring, academic patient has come here in an attempt to share his journey and also make it interesting for the reader by trying to make the current account less of an academic rant and more of a personal experience. At the very outset, I must say that the quote by Friedrich Engels shouldn't make you think that this chapter is a tribute to Marx's close aide and companion. Rather, it is an epiphany on the importance of the family in the life of a Left-baptized academic who had developed an attitude of disdain, similar to that of Engels towards the "institution of family." While the above quote about family as an oppressive structure for women might appear true even in our times, yet at the risk of being "canceled" again by Marxists for my heresy, this chapter is dedicated to the newfound value of family, friends, and most importantly, my guru in my life. I discovered this value during the crisis I faced over the past two years. This is a story of rediscovery of the importance of familial bonds and society at a time when the pre-cancer author had become cynical of these as outdated relics of the past.

This chapter deliberately begins with a Sanskrit sloka dedicated to the guru or teacher. On further examination, the Sanskrit word "guru" can be further broken down into *gu* or darkness and *ru* or remover. Taken together, a guru is the "remover of darkness" or the one who removes the darkness of ignorance by bringing in the light of knowledge. In my cancer journey, it was my guru my professor at Ashoka University, whose vital support and words of wisdom redeemed me from the quagmire of hopelessness and darkness I was getting trapped into after hearing about my diagnosis in March 2021. It was his words heard via a Zoom meeting that came as a ray of hope and prevented me from being engulfed by darkness. Hence, by beginning the chapter with the sloka dedicated to the guru, the following pages pay a tribute to him as well as to my parents, family, and friends—in other words, society.

My guru gave me the first rope of hope to hold on to by stating that it was not an accident, but an opportunity to learn and inculcate the values of perseverance, courage, and determination bestowed upon me by the Divine (elaborated in a later chapter). He acted like the pole star whose brightness helped the ship of my life sail through the turbulent waters I found myself in. After diagnosis, once the initial weeks at the hospital passed, the next pressing issue was finding a suitable place to stay in the city for the next 10 or 12 odd months. With the help of my uncle, we found a flat in faraway Noida, but the only drawback was the distance between the flat and the hospital. It would take around two hours via car on a traffic-free day. As we (especially I) were adjusting to the idea of having to stay away in a remote corner of some concrete jungle (Delhi was much greener, comparatively), the visit by my Guruji accompanied by some of my classmates from Ashoka University resembled the arrival of a fresh cool breeze in a desert. The cool breeze was my Guruji's request for me and my parents to stay at his house in Vasant Kunj, a posh area in South Delhi, which was a far better option than the exile in Noida. Not only did he voluntarily offer his own house but also sought no rent. He even offered to pay the expenses of food, water, gas, and electricity; however, my parents and I insisted on paying the latter expenses as we would be the ones to avail those services. Honestly speaking, the offer left us flabbergasted ("surprise" would not suffice to capture our emotions back then) as it was not only unexpected, but also shattered the various myths and pre-conceptions we had about "Delhi-wallahs"— aggressive, loud-mouthed, scheming, and cunning lot who were on the lookout to dupe "innocent" strangers like us. In the 21st century *Kaliyuga* (the last stage of the Hindu time cycle after *Satya, Treta,* and *Dwapar Yugas*), one would be considered a fool for even offering to pay the electricity and water bills for another, and that too in an expensive city like Delhi. Yet, there was Guruji, with his *karuna* (kindness) right at the time when we needed it.

In the days to come, Guruji's karuna was seen in many other ways. Just like in the sloka quoted at the beginning of the chapter, Guruji would play the role of the Holy Trinity of Hinduism by first creating within me the hope of survival and recovery before I came to Delhi (Brahma), then with his kindness, charity, constant support, he preserved and boosted my willpower to recover (Vishnu), and it was his words and advice that erased the pessimism and hopelessness within me (Shiva). In addition, he has been like the ever-present Brahma, supporting me in every stage of the journey till date, through weekly meetings, phone calls, mails, and Zoom conferences. Not only did he give us shelter but he even took the lead in organizing a fundraising campaign for me on Milaap along with my cousin and friends from Ashoka University. Additionally, he also sought out high-income donors among his networks and donated a considerable sum to the campaign. The debt I owe to Guruji increased again in the first half of 2022 when my parents and I were gripped with the dilemma of whether we had overstayed his hospitality or imposed too much on his kindness. Having heard our concerns, he laughed and plainly said, "This is your home as well. Stay here until you are healed."

I think it would take me seven lifetimes to repay Guruji's karuna and gyan or give him a *gurudakshina* (an offering made to the guru in return for their guidance). Though at first, I only knew him as a teacher, post my diagnosis he became my guru who taught me the values of courage, self-confidence, and generosity not only through e-mails and Zoom meetings but also through his actions. At this point, I should stop praising my Guruji as continuing to do so would turn this chapter into a ballad or *mahakavya* (epic poetry) of the yore.

The next on the dedication list are my parents. Throughout this ordeal, both my parents have been like two strong pillars that have supported the shaky foundations of my life. Although we have been together since my birth, it was only after my diagnosis that I got the opportunity to witness the extent of their inner strength and determination. I cannot imagine acting with such strength had I been in their place.

During the crisis, my father appeared to me as the epitome of stoicism. He did not budge even an inch under the tremendous amount of pressure, especially when I, with my comorbidities, was at high risk during the horrific second wave of COVID-19 in 2021 as well as the 21-day solitary confinement period during my Bone Marrow Transplant (BMT) in September of the same year. Despite my descent into hopelessness, he never lost heart even for a moment and always urged me to carry on. It was no wonder that in March 2022, the head doctor remarked to me, "Your father stood like a pillar with you throughout a year and more. Never forget that." My mother played an equally important part by providing her vital support to both of us. If my father was the pillar in my journey through the world of "secular medicine," my mother played the same in my "spiritual healing." From the initial "divine sign" at the Sai Baba Temple in Delhi (to be elaborated on in my next chapter) to traveling frequently to Haridwar to perform a *havan* on my behalf, she was always praying for my recovery. Even now, she routinely donates in my name. However, I must admit I sometimes get irritated with her when I see her religiosity transforming into an obsession. Both of my parents, together with my Guruji, have played the role of *Trideva* or the Hindu Trinity in my life. No wonder my uncle had remarked "Your parents are your Gods now. Worship them throughout your life."

This entire experience changed my perspective about the relationship I had with my parents. While in my earlier undergraduate days, armed with the new academic theories drilled into our heads regarding society and family, I regarded them as mere blind followers of age-old orthodox values, my views changed completely on seeing my parents stick with me throughout this ordeal without a moment's rest. It only seemed to reinforce their often-said words that it is family that matters in the end. The strength required to write this chapter is owed to them as it was their presence and constant support that improved my mental and physical health to the extent that I am able to type down these pages.

Last but not least, this experience made me realize the value of the extended family or cousins and kin, as well as that of friends, both current as well as long-lost ones. Our initial stay and my treatment in Delhi would not have been possible without the staunch and unfailing support of my *Khura and Khuri* (uncle and aunt in Assamese) and their son. It was my Khura who accompanied and helped us financially in the time of our greatest need. Not only that, when my father had to run from pillar to post searching for blood donors, it was my uncle who not only donated blood at the hospital but also requested his colleagues and subordinates to do the same. In addition, my cousin and his friend volunteered to donate blood for my sake, even without my asking. My aunt not only supported my mother in the initial days of my admittance but also started seeking "spiritual medicine" for my sake with my mother. Without the presence of my uncle's family in Delhi, it would have been impossible for us to achieve any stability or firm footing to deal with the crisis. Hence, my dad would often say that uncle's transfer from Mumbai to Delhi just a year before my illness was a part of the divine plan. Along with my uncle, my entire extended family came together to see us through the crisis, be it in the form of financial help and spiritual help (prayers and donations in holy places for my recovery), or by providing emotional and mental support through frequent calls and advice. Most importantly, they never allowed us to lose hope or go down the abyss.

Equally important were my friends—batchmates and juniors as well as teachers from Ashoka University—who came together to provide emotional, mental, and, most importantly financial support. They organized a concert to raise funds for me and a junior who was also facing a similar crisis. Their efforts reduced the burden upon my parents to a large extent, as it covered a significant part of the cost including the payment made to my bone marrow donor. In the immediate years post my graduating from Ashoka, I had become skeptical of phrases often brought up in the inaugural orientation such as the "Ashoka Family," "Ashoka Fraternity", or the motto of the Young India Fellowship PG Diploma program, "The fellowship never ends." Given my previous experiences of farewell promises of "keeping in touch" after school and college which had not lasted for very long, I had similar expectations from Ashoka as well. But, even after two years, the entire "Ashoka family" mobilized to support me and my parents during the most challenging times. Looking back, I can confidently say that the fellowship actually never ends. It comes back to help you emerge from the quagmire of cynicism when you least expect it.

People like my cousins and my classmates whom I had thought to be distant entities, busy in the humdrum of their own lives, came to my rescue in the time of crisis. This forced me to change my earlier perception of the society and social cohesion as nothing but illusory terms in the current rat race of the 21st century. The help and support extended by my kin and friends made me see friendship and kinship in a new light as bonds that, despite being submerged deep in the schedules and time tables of the globalized world, surface in unexpected ways to help and support each other. Friendships and kinship ties do not necessarily require the performance of monthly or weekly calls as a ritual. It might be enough to reach out at the right time when one is in dire need of social support and aid.

I think it is time for me to stop here because if I were to list down and acknowledge the contribution of all, the chapter would rival the combined size of Homer's *Iliad* and *Odyssey*. Such is the level of indebtedness and gratitude I find myself in. I believe the cancer experience was a part of the divine plan for me in order to make me realize the vital need of society, regardless of the theories and ideas brandished in political science or sociology classes in most universities. I am tempted to quote Foucault's title "Society must be defended." Though, unlike the Leftist thinker, I'd like to believe in the literal meaning. I would like to say that society must be defended as we, *Homo sapiens*, are social animals and will always be. Especially for us Asians, our existence and identity will inevitably include the *parivaar* (family), *kutumb* (kin), *and qaum* (community) that encompasses the entire world. Or else why would the ancient sages say *Vasudaiva kutumbakam* (the entire world is one family)?

—Anuraag Khaund

MANAGING
MENTAL HEALTH

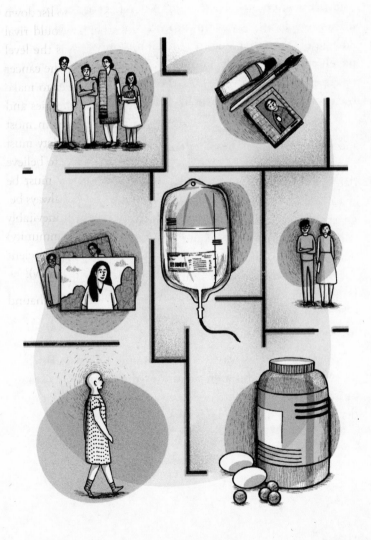

Cancer affects your physical health in obvious, visible ways, but it also wreaks havoc on your mental and emotional health in insidious ways. Right from the time you are diagnosed, you go through the motions, one foot in front of the other, as per your treatment protocol with no time to reflect or analyze. No matter how long or short this process is, if you are lucky, you emerge on the other side in remission, tumor-free, or completely cured. A few unlucky ones are stuck with maintenance or experimental treatments. At the end of active treatment, the enormity of it all hits you like a ton of bricks.

Many think the physical effects of the treatment are the most difficult part of the experience. However, post-treatment mental health issues can be equally challenging, if not more debilitating. During your active treatment, you don't have the space, time, or mental bandwidth to think about anything apart from getting through it all. But later, you are overcome with emotions, mainly grief and sadness. You ask yourself several questions—Why me? What caused it? Is this *karma* or *kismet*? You mourn the loss of your pre-cancer self—your dreams, hopes, aspirations, health, and well-being that you may have taken for granted. You start rebuilding your new post-cancer identity from scratch.

They say youth is wasted on the young. I'd say health is wasted on those who aren't aware of their mortality. Read on to discover how some of our co-authors dealt with or are dealing with similar mental battles.

THE MIND GAME

Act 1: The Fall

"The doctor has recommended that you bring your husband for the appointment," said the receptionist.

"What? Why?" I asked quizzically.

"She has recommended," the receptionist repeated.

Now, I have always believed that I am a strong, independent woman, who can handle her own problems, so the receptionist's words did not sit well with me. But I just sighed. New country, new rules, I thought.

So, on a Friday afternoon, battling anxiety and confusion, while also filled with disdain for the "bring your husband" request, I marched into the doctor's office, with my husband in tow.

The last time I had been to her clinic there had been a small painting on the wall. It was no longer there. I looked around imagining how I would have restyled the room to make it more warm and inviting. Maybe a few plants here and there, and that beautiful painting I had seen at the art gallery the other day would work well. And that's when I heard the words.

"The mass, which we sent for biopsy, is unfortunately cancerous..."

You see, right there in that moment, when most people would go into complete shock, my mind flashed a scene from the Bollywood movie *Anand*.

When the doctor tells the main protagonist, *"You have lymphosarcoma of the intestine,"* basically a terminal disease, he walks off into the sunset, humming beautiful sad songs. In my drama queen of a mind, I was Anand, and I saw myself walk to God-knows-where, humming medley of sad songs that were already spinning in my head.

That was my introduction to the disease which would consume me for the next two years and counting.

Honestly, I don't remember much of what happened next. It was just a battery of tests, visits to doctors, search for the right oncologist, insurance, and more.

"Hopefully, we have caught it early," my husband said, as we were heading to the doctor to know the results of the PET scan.

I shrugged. Hope was the last thing I felt. Anger, self-pity, fear maybe, but not hope for sure.

It was agonizing stepping into her clinic a week later. My mind was racing, and I kept staring at the report in front of her, willing it to be good. I was also chanting a prayer to calm my frayed nerves.

"It is metastatic. It has gone into your lungs, liver, and the bone..."

Well, so much for hoping.

As the doctor continued, a number flashed before my eyes: 25%. That was the approximate chance that research was giving me of surviving beyond five years. *Wow, I am Anand!*

It almost felt like someone had punched me hard in the gut. I was 37, married for three years to my childhood best friend; I had moved countries recently (India to Singapore), and had our first baby four months back. My life that finally seemed to be coming together was now blowing up in my face.

As the shock wore off over the next few weeks, I felt a guttural scream stuck inside me. The same I had felt when my mother had died, earlier that year. I could not say goodbye to her because my pregnancy prevented me from traveling back to India. I couldn't even cry, for I feared harming my unborn child.

This same scream seemed to be stuck inside me again.

Why me? Why me? My silent shrieks would fill my head while my calm façade gave nothing away. I prided myself on how calmly I was able to inform my father.

"Dad, I have Stage 4, breast cancer. We are to immediately begin treatment. Don't worry, everything is under control."

That was great Snehal, keep it up. No one needs to know how you feel.

Act 2: Sinking Quickly

Soon my chemotherapy was in full swing, and I felt a darkness creeping inside. My thoughts wouldn't leave me alone. It was almost as if I derived some masochistic pleasure holding onto these dark thoughts.

Slowly, my hair began to fall. Every morning I would find clumps of hair on my pillow, and I would gulp back tears. My skin lost its healthy glow and looked sallow. When I looked in the mirror every day, I saw myself transforming into someone I did not know.

Mirror, mirror on the wall, who is the ugliest of them all?

"I think I look like Smeagol (the pale, sickly-looking creature from *Lord of the Rings*)," I told my husband one morning. We both laughed. Well, at least the cancer hadn't destroyed my sense of humor.

I hated how I looked. I hated how I felt. People tell you to love your body through cancer. But how can you love a body you barely recognize?

But the worst fear I was dealing with was the what-will-people-say syndrome.

I believed I had learned to deal with this dark cloud when I divorced my ex-husband. But sadly, I hadn't, and the cloud got heavier every time I decided to step out. What would people say when they saw me? Would they judge me? Call me weak? Would they be afraid of me?

I stopped stepping out, stopped taking my kid to the park. I wasn't strong enough to face people. The only place I visited regularly was the temple. God was the only reason I would risk facing public scrutiny. I thanked my stars that I wasn't working then, and that I wasn't in India where I might have had to face the brutally sympathetic and curious questions and glances of people I knew.

All our life we are told to be strong. I was exceptionally good at maintaining that front. *Vulnerability is for the weak*, I thought. But right now, there were chinks in my armor. Though I wanted to be a warrior princess, I couldn't help being Moaning Myrtle (from the *Harry Potter* series).

"If you want to leave me, I will understand," I told my husband one day.

No, I won't understand! I will probably die, and my ghost will come back and haunt you for a long time!

"I'm not going to leave you, Snehal," he sighed. He was getting used to my melodrama.

I would often wonder what it would take for him to leave me. Would he get tired of my disease or me first? What would happen to my son Samar after I was gone? Who would love him and dote on him? I almost started waiting for people around me to say they were done with me.

I went into a shell. I did not meet people; I did not want to talk to anyone. I had officially become a recluse. Miserable, afraid, and lonely.

The worst part was that my treatment progressed like a roller-coaster ride. Each time we thought it would work, the cancer would rear its head. And then the treatment plan would change to something stronger, leaving me weaker and unhappier.

I would see people put up their remission pictures, and I would often wonder when I would put up mine. I had chosen a dress for the occasion, too, the first time we thought I was cancer free. It still hangs in my closet.

So much was resting on that day. My future, my career. I saw all my ex-colleagues and friends moving on with their life, their work, and their family while I seemed to be stuck in some sort of a time warp.

I was waiting to restart life. Reboot my career. Select all and delete what had happened to me in the last several months and start afresh. But as the days wore on and with no respite in sight, I slowly started sinking.

Act 3: The Game!

My aunt Vrushali is one of the most carefree women I have met. A doctor by profession, she always has a refreshing take on any problem I am mulling over. In a sense, she is quite the role model for me.

"Snehal, cancer is a mind game!" she said, while I was sharing updates about my treatment plan.

So, I'm not the only one losing it here. What did that even mean? Cancer is spreading all through my body here, and she says the game is being played in my head?

By this time, I had reached one of the lowest points in my life. My thoughts were spiraling out of control.

Through the blur, I knew that I was debilitating myself more than my illness demanded. The vicious beliefs I had developed were so strong that my feeble attempts at reining them in were proving futile.

I think many of us carry such beliefs, in varying degrees. But we take notice only when they start crippling us.

I could see how my darkness was impacting the people I loved. I saw my husband aging faster than ever. I saw my little one crawl to me and hug me, maybe sensing my sadness. I could see my family praying fervently to God. I could see my friends struggling to find the right words to say to me.

I wanted to change things, make them better for me and the people I loved. My aunt's words echoed in my head. But I just did not know what to do.

Belief 1: I Don't Need Help!

"Can we talk?" Suruchi asked quietly.

"I don't need counseling, Suruchi," I sighed.

"I just want to talk. Nothing else," she urged. Suruchi was my close friend since we were 16 years old and was now a trained counselor.

"I don't need help. I am fine," I stated firmly.

It wasn't only her; I was pushing away everyone I truly loved, those who wanted nothing else but to be there for me. I feared they were helping me out of sympathy.

But Suruchi could be persuasive. Thus began our journey together.

And we spoke a lot, but not so much about cancer. We spoke about my life, my relationships, my emotions, and so much more. Slowly, she helped me unpack all my emotional baggage and deal with it in a way that was healthy. She helped me heal from traumas of the past such as my divorce and my mother's death. One of my biggest victories was that I finally accepted I had cancer. So far, my game plan had been denial and distraction.

As this journey continued, I gradually became comfortable seeking help from others. I needed the help, and I realized that far from making me feel weak, it enabled me to face my challenges from a position of strength.

Belief 2: People Are Judging Me!

In our sessions, we covered some of my other fears as well that I seemed to have happily nurtured through cancer.

"I can't go out, they will judge me," I said.

"Who will?" she asked.

"The people on the road, in my condominium, anyone I know," I shrieked.

"And how will they judge you?" she asked.

"They will call me weak, they will be scared of me," I retorted.

"Have you heard them call you weak or being afraid of you the few times you met them?" she asked again.

"No, not really," I shrugged.

"Are you judging yourself, or are they? And even if they call you weak, would it make you weak?"

So, I slowly started stepping out, staring at people to confirm my fears. And then it happened. The stare came from a passenger in the metro. I looked and then looked away, but she continued staring. Then she got up and came to me. I nearly stopped breathing as she sat near me and gently asked, "I'm not trying to be rude, but are you suffering from cancer or some other disease?"

I sputtered, "Cancer."

See this is what I was talking about. She is judging me! I knew I shouldn't have stepped out! I knew it... I...

"My sister died from cancer last year," she said. "I just want to wish you all the strength and love," she whispered and left.

It took me a minute to find my bearings and breathe again. And then the tears rolled down.

People can be kind, I guess!

Belief 3: I Don't Have Anything to Be Grateful For!

As the days passed, I started noticing that my mind was at loggerheads with herself. She would constantly contradict herself. The nervous little Smeagol that she had become, alone in her cave with her "precious" thoughts, was now voicing contrasting opinions.

I don't have anything to be grateful for! I got cancer... at 37... when my baby was just four months old! Life is unfair, unfair!

Is there nothing to be grateful for?

No!

Snehal, you have the best medical facilities at your disposal. A loving husband and a beautiful, healthy child. Your in-laws have pretty much stopped their life for you, to help you raise Samar. Your circle of friends is there for you, no matter what. Do you want me to say more? While God has been unkind, he has also given you so much to overcome this challenge!

Silence!

Whoa! Where did that come from?

And that one exchange, in a way, changed how I perceived my situation. I slowly started noticing the silver lining in every cloud. I stopped feeling like a victim with the constant blame game in my head.

I started journaling my gratitude every night. I might have laughed it off earlier in my life, but it was a saving grace for me at that time, and to this day.

Belief 4: I Can't Do Anything Till I'm Cancer-free!

But with eight months of treatment, and my cancer still behaving like a game of whack-a-mole, I remember a particularly dark day.

I was sobbing and cursing my fate, when my husband looked at me and said, "Don't let life stop, Snehal. You keep telling me about the things you want to do once you are cancer-free, but what stops you now? You have two weeks between every chemo session when you are fine. Why don't you try something?"

What the hell is happening to people around me? Why is everyone turning into Sadhguru? It's particularly irritating when he is right!

But to tell you the truth, that was one big "light-bulb" moment for me. You know, it's so natural to be drawn inward that when he shone the torch externally, it suddenly made me realize that my life could have a purpose beyond recovery. Something on which I could refocus my energy. Something that would help me find more meaning in my everyday life.

Belief 5: I Have No Future!

"I was hoping to reinitiate my coaching journey but I'm not sure if my treatment will allow for the rigor the certification needs," I said shakily to my mentor.

I had begun training to be a Life & Career Coach almost five years ago, and I had enjoyed the experience. But somehow, I did not complete the program.

Now, as I struggled to understand where to begin, I thought of reaching out to my mentor. Someone I had worked with and highly respected during my professional days.

"Don't worry, Snehal. We will do it," he said calmly.

He thinks I can. My husband thinks I can. Can I?

With that, I slowly re-entered the world of coaching. My small computer screen (this was during the time of the pandemic, when everything was happening online) allowed me to discover a unique, beautiful world, almost like the one in the movie *Avatar*.

I met wonderful coaches along the way who became part of my tribe. I worked with some amazing clients, sharing a truly symbiotic relationship in which I was discovering as much about myself as about them.

Coaching energized me. It made me happy. I had finally found my passion!

And then one day, out of the blue, I discovered cancer advocacy. I had been thinking about sharing my story. I honestly don't know what I was expecting would be the outcome. I only knew I wanted to reach out to others, those with similar stories, and let them know they were not alone.

That's when I got my first opportunity with a media house.

Now the world will know, Snehal. You can't hide anymore.

After the piece came out, many people wrote to me; some who needed hope, some who wanted to give hope, and others who had seen their loved ones suffer.

It was overwhelming yet wonderful to be able to contribute, even in a small way. It made me realize that I wanted to continue this dialogue and reach out to more people.

I would also keep scouring the comments section for words such as "weak," "poor thing," or "tragedy" but there were none.

Finally, I had started getting a foothold on life again. I started seeing a future for myself. I was changing course and becoming a different version of me, someone who my treatment would be kind to. But the best part was that I was slowly learning to love this person and love the unchartered territories she was entering.

Act 4: Where Am I Now?

I still live with cancer, but I am not here to wage a war against it. It's too much aggression in my head. I just want to heal. Heal my body, heal my mind, and be proud of who I am becoming.

I have learned to just trust my journey. Cancer brought me to my knees and made me understand this life lesson. So, I'm taking it one day at a time.

I am a work-in-progress, pretty much like everyone else. I am still discovering this new Snehal. I have my good days and bad; days I want to be a hermit and days I want to socialize. But overall, I have learned to respect the fragility of life and what it brings my way.

See, we are all told to "live each day like it is your last," "don't take life for granted," and so on. But some of us get a knock on our head to truly experience its essence.

Ouch! Too much drama? But I am a drama queen!

So, this is where I conclude. I'll leave you with a poem that pretty much sums up what my journey was like in my first year of treatment.

And I bid adieu to one of the most perplexing years of my life,

A year I thought would be a battle turned out to be a year of quiet reflection.

A year I thought would be full of hiding and going into my shell turned out to be a year of full disclosure and self-love.

A year I thought would be a long wait for the end turned out to be a year of trusting my journey.

A year I thought would be debilitating turned out to be a year of meeting my passion.

Today, say a little prayer and thank the universe for all that you have learned through strife or love.

There is more to come; the waves of life will always be there.

But that is their beauty; if not for the turbulence, how can we learn to admire the calm?

Have a glorious year end and a happy new year!

—Snehal Ponde

WHO AM I?

Does the term "Ship of Theseus" sound familiar? I first learned about the "Ship of Theseus" dilemma in my philosophy class in 2014. It has captivated me ever since. According to a Greek legend, the ship that had carried Theseus and the young people of Athens when they returned from Crete, had thirty oars. The oars were gradually replaced with new ones until all of them were brand new. The paradox raises the question: whether this ship, all of whose components have been changed, can still be considered the same ship.

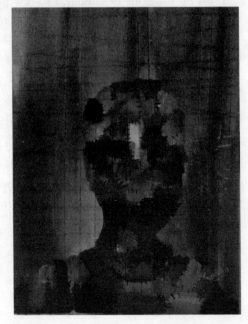

I found it so amusing at the time that I painted it as I saw this dilemma in real life. Who would have imagined that almost eight years later our paths would converge in such a profound way that I would examine my life's experiences through the lens of this paradox?

On my 29th birthday, I was peppy, motivated, in love with my life, and optimistic about a bright future with my beloved husband and future kids. That day, I prayed in the morning, dressed in bright pink, left my long brown hair open, wore the new pair of earrings my husband had gifted, and went to work happily. The whole day passed in an instant, anticipating the evening dinner planned with family, friends, and some colleagues my husband had invited. I was doing great at work, was excited about an upcoming vacation, and had my parents visiting me for my birthday. What else could I possibly ask for?

That evening, I recall, I began by introducing myself to my husband's colleagues by stating my name, followed by my work description. If someone continued to show interest, I told them about my personal interests and perhaps shared a few anecdotes about my hometown in India.

After over two years of my stint as a mother with cancer, that introduction remains the same.

If I meet someone new today, I start with my name, followed by my job profile (even my job profile hasn't changed in this time). Then, if someone shows more interest, like before, I talk about my hobbies and maybe a few stories about the place I am from in India.

If our identities are determined by how we introduce ourselves to others, then, for me, hardly anything has changed. And yet, when I look in the mirror deep into my eyes, I struggle to find who I am today.

Am I that peppy girl who was in a happy marriage, excited about life and the many adventures it had to offer? Or am I the realistic, solid woman who has become unabashed by the difficult journey of navigating motherhood and cancer with limited support?

If I'm that ship from the paradox, and if my body and mind have changed after cancer, am I even myself? Who is Thanisha? I often wonder.

I find myself oscillating between the past and the present, caught up in the loop of who I was, what I've become, and which parts of my present self I want to take forward with me. This choice constantly burdens me as some parts of me are dead and the new ones are too new. It is like living a new life but still holding onto my old life. It's like being reborn without dying.

Motherhood Interrupted

One of the first things I lost from the life I had pictured for myself was the kind of motherhood I had imagined.

During my pregnancy, I had made plans of what I would do after giving birth. I fully intended to cherish my maternity leave to bond with my newborn, learn the new mama chops, and use the downtime to relax. I wanted to go for the many cocktails and Thai massages I missed during pregnancy. A part of me was hoping there would be time to do a part-time MBA on the side while following a rigorous exercise and diet routine to get back in shape. I always told myself I didn't want to be an out-of-shape mommy.

My diagnosis distorted those plans. I had to prepare myself for a strenuous treatment that required me to spend numerous hours in the hospital, with side effects that would hinder my weight loss goals and cause my energy levels to dip, which would limit me from bonding with my baby. Motherhood looked very different from what I had imagined it to be.

Even today, it's hard for me to think about the early months of motherhood without getting caught up in memories of the dark times I spent shuttling between the hospital and home. I spent many hours waiting alone in billing queues which I could have spent playing with my son.

Losing My Physical Self: One Bit at a Time

I remember it was after the second chemo session that my hair started to fall and I decided to shave off my head completely. I asked my then nanny to use my husband's electric shaver to get rid of every bit of my hair. While I tried to put on a brave face on seeing my silky locks fall on the ground, the way my near and dear ones reacted made me feel profound misery and shame.

I still remember the well-rounded naked head was a surprise for my husband and family. I had imagined them looking at me with eyes full of love. I wanted them to tell me how it didn't change the wonderful person I was.

On the contrary, their first reaction was as if they were seeing an ugly blobfish. Remembering how terrible I felt that day still sends chills through my spine. Losing my long golden-brown soft and silky locks was more difficult than I had imagined. It was like losing a part of who I was, the comforting face I always saw in the mirror.

Soon after, my body started experiencing other side effects. Low stamina, breathlessness, inflamed stomach, venous thrombosis, and extreme pains from peripheral neuropathy limited my physical abilities. My plans of celebrating my 30th birthday by running a half marathon took a backseat.

From the "Most Happening Girl" to the One with Social Anxiety

When I entered the first year of undergraduate college, our seniors had hosted a fresher's party. I had dressed up in a black fit-and-flare dress, styled my long hair in a half tie, and just owned the dance floor that night. I had danced with almost everyone and had been beaming with a smile throughout the night.

That night, I hadn't been announced "Miss Freshers." However, the hosts had introduced a new title on the spot to crown me the "Most Happening Girl." That had been me in 2008.

Fast forward to 2020, sometime after my fourth chemo, I started disliking talking to people entirely. Whenever I would speak to someone, it would mean repeating the whole story about my diagnosis and motherhood, followed by a response that was either pity or toxic positivity. I was tired of hearing people say "sorry," "don't worry, things are not too bad," or "things will just be fine."

I was so tired that I started to shell up. Sometimes I wanted to yell out for help and support, but I began to be reserved because it seemed too daunting to talk to someone. The idea that I would have to pick up the phone and call someone on their birthday or anniversary gave me sleepless nights. On my own birthday, I wished my phone battery would die so I could respond later to people via a message.

That "Most Happening Girl" had become someone who got anxiety attacks around people. Hopefully, someday the peppy part of me will come alive again.

The Divine Plan

My mom is a regular temple-goer. She will tell you that she got into that habit because of me. Her tryst with temple visits started because the 10-year-old me wanted to go to the temple every Tuesday, and she was the only one around to drop me.

I had always believed there's a divine plan and everything happens for a good reason. With this attitude, life had been easier to navigate. I always thought someone was looking out for me.

When cancer struck me, I used my spiritual side to navigate the treatment. But after every hospital visit, I started to doubt the existence of any such divine plan. My mind mulled on, "Why me?" While I have made my peace with cancer, I don't think it left me with any faith in the divine plan. Every day feels more operational, less divine; every night feels long and sleepless. I'm constantly struggling to find the peace I once had.

Losing "Home"

One of the most significant losses has been the loss of "home." Home for me has never been a structure made out of bricks; it has always been the people with whom I feel like I belong. It's a sentiment.

In 2020, as we awaited our soon-to-be-born child, I lived my fairytale life with my husband in Bangkok. I was the happy single child of my parents, who adored me and were my most reliable confidants. But cancer made me feel like my home was slipping away from my hands because my relationships with those dearest to me changed.

Lost Innocence

When I was diagnosed with cancer, my parents were in denial for some time. They kept hoping and suggesting that my diagnosis was wrong. They believed it had something to do with my pregnancy, and it would subside after I delivered the baby. It was understandably hard for my parents to deal with the fact that their only daughter, who was pregnant for the first time, had become a cancer patient.

It took them a long time to accept and be my comforting safe space again. During that prolonged period, I created a shell around me retreating deeper and deeper within myself. The child within me who always relied on her folks for emotional strength was lost. The part of me that made me feel most safe and at home no longer existed.

Even though today my parents are back to being my pillars of strength, the cracks from the ordeal have changed me forever. Maybe, I've seen too much in the past two years, and it's just hard to be that innocent child to my parents again.

From Fairytales to Reality

It's always shown in movies that marriage is a commitment in which one has to be constantly there for the other in times of need. Often, the hero or the heroine will either fall sick or get trapped in a mess and the other partner will prioritize taking care of the latter above everything else. When I got married, perhaps like everyone else, I too thought I could count on my partner to fetch the moon for me if needed.

Cancer came in hard on my companionship. It was something my partner and I had to cope with in our way. It made me see the extent of my needs and the hole I could feel when my partner wouldn't be as available as I needed.

I've been alone so often during the past two years that I've lost count. There have been too many solo hospital visits, struggles to find and train nannies, and many nights of pain and care for our baby. There were so many times I wanted someone to accompany me when I had to visit the hospital or to sit with me later to remind me how special I was to them. But there I was, feeling lonely to the bone.

We had many conversations, but the responses left me stranded. And the many conversations we didn't have created a gap too wide to cover only with optimism. People may call me demanding or needy, but for me, the needs I had from my relationship changed from wanting a secure future to the desire for a more peaceful and intimate present. The future is too far and unpredictable for me. So, I look for warmth today instead of hoping for an unknown tomorrow.

While things have improved slowly over the last few months, the scars that the two years have left on my companionship sometimes seem too hard to heal. My heart often mourns over the ghosts of the dreamer in me who fantasized about a fairytale life. Sometimes it feels like I'm at a crossroad where the romantic Thanisha of the past keeps competing with the realistic and pragmatic Thanisha of today.

While I still believe in love and dote my son unconditionally, the affectionate relationship I once shared with my husband now seems worn out. The time I spend with my son brings me joy and happiness, but the distance I see in my other relationships reminds me of the unmet needs and expectations I once had. It constantly takes me to the times I was heartbroken and found myself alone and miserable. It makes me feel hopeless.

I struggle to see the light at the end of the tunnel and find my way back home again. Perhaps, someday I will be able to take the broken pieces of my heart and join them back. Then, finally, I may have a place again, a feeling I can call "home."

What (Really) Matters

Once in college I had lied to a friend about not having access to a past year's quiz. Later, she had found out, and our relationship was never the same. Fast forward to 2019. I negotiated a promotion at my company based on a competing offer. I rejected a job offer at a firm where I could have potentially learned more because they offered me a lower title. I was the youngest "Director of Product" I knew, and this mattered much more than spending time reflecting on what brought me peace. I remember I was so sure about the notion of a working mom that, at times, I ridiculed and misjudged at-home moms. I was this ambitious working woman running the race of titles and growth. It was hard to let go of the carrot of a rich, luxurious life in the future.

The journey through cancer has changed me. It has made me realize the unpredictability of life. I've experienced my deepest fears and worst nightmares. While there were moments of weakness when I wanted to quit and die, it was during this time that I've been at my strongest. This time has transformed my principles and things that matter to me. It has made me more interested in knowing someone for who they are rather than their job titles. Rather than pretending to be perfect, I'm much more comfortable with being just myself, as imperfect as I might be. I'm much more comfortable saying no to things that I don't want to do. I'm more aware of what brings me happiness, and I want to do it over other things every single day.

Rather than building a fortune for my son and imagining his graduation from Oxford or Harvard, I make it a point to spend quality time with him daily. I don't know how long I'll live to be able to do this. So, I prioritize calling my parents daily, visiting them every few months, and being there for the people who matter to me.

What Will the Ship Say?

When I take a step back, I often wonder what the ship from the paradox would say if it had a soul and a voice. I don't think it would stop to consider whether it is the same ship or not. It might be more interested in telling stories about the pieces that were lost and sharing its feelings about the loss. Perhaps it would like to talk about the new pieces. Or maybe it would talk about the fears it has or the struggles it deals with.

Looking at my life through this paradox, my basic introduction and physical identity have barely changed over time. Yet, my beliefs about life, relationships, faith, and value systems are poles apart from what they were two years ago. I often wonder if the chemo-therapy drugs in my blood, the tiny marks from the biopsy, the burden of the unmet expectations I had from my loved ones, and the lack of support from them have scarred me permanently.

When I look for that peppy, ambitious, optimistic, romantic girl, I only find shadows.

The ship of my life mourns the loss of the past. And the newness of the present gives it jitters. It often feels lonely, depressed, and broken. It is afraid of how the travelers will perceive it. Will they expect it to be the same ship? Will they be repulsed by the changes and retire it to the docks?

The ship struggles with its many imperfections, yet it hopes to find a way to move on. It aspires to be able to embrace the changes it has undergone. It longs for the travelers who will one day share their journeys with it and lovingly accept it for what it is. It hopes to go to far-flung places eventually and see all that the world has to offer before retiring peacefully.

—Thanisha Sehgal

MAINTAINING PHYSICAL WELL-BEING

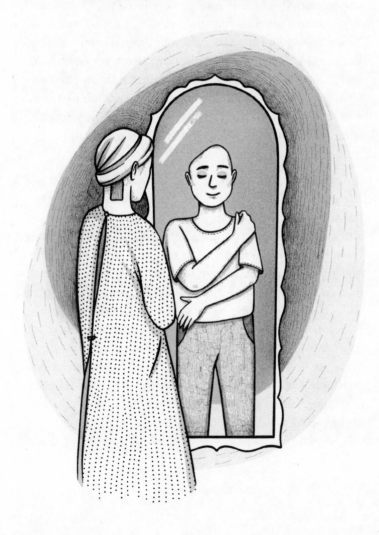

Recouping from the assault that cancer and its treatment inflicts on your body takes a long time. The process means different things to different people. It could mean growing out or shaving your hair, losing or regaining your weight, and rehabilitating or rebuilding your strength, stamina, and confidence. It could mean revamping your lifestyle completely and becoming a person who eats healthy, sleeps for eight hours every night, and exercises regularly. Adjusting to this new routine might take months, sometimes even years. You try to find a routine that works for you, instead of comparing yourself to what cancer muggles (non-cancer folks) are able to do.

Despite your efforts, your body might never go back to its pre-cancer self. You may have to make peace with this fact and live with your impediments. So, you do what you can and learn to love your body for what it has endured to keep you alive. On rainy days, you might still feel insecure about your body, but you try to find ways to feel good in your own skin. You try to be compassionate with yourself when you cheat once in a while to eat your favorite food or sleep in instead of going for that morning walk. Your post-cancer life becomes a life of moderation. After all this, you still may often ask yourself, what's the point of being alive or living longer if you don't get to do the things you like, right? Read these stories of people like you who are dealing with their own physical challenges. Each of them found their own ways to take care of themselves.

THE WEIGHT OF WORDS

"**I** need to be fit again, but I don't know where to begin," I said to my sister.

"I want to own my appearance and not be defined by cancer," I said to my fiancé.

Conversations like this play in my mind when I recall my journey of dealing with weight gain, hair loss, and all the other physical tolls that cancer takes on our bodies, and we involuntarily accept. Six months of chemotherapy had left me feeling weak and sluggish. My wedding was just a few months away. I wanted to regain my stamina and feel fit. I was racing against time to fit comfortably in my wedding outfits. Like any other bride, I wanted to look the best version of myself on my wedding day.

I had not been active and did not have an exercise routine while I was on treatment, but I was eager to jump right in and start. The harsh chemotherapy regime had disrupted my appetite. I was unable to eat well on treatment days, but I craved to eat good food once I felt better. I aspired to strike a balance between eating healthy and being able to enjoy tasty foods after recovering. In addition, I had become extremely conscious about gaining weight due to chemotherapy, as we approached my wedding date.

Chemotherapy had already caused hair loss. Post treatment, seeing my hair grow again, although slowly, was comforting. The growth rate of my hair was not within my control but becoming fit and improving my stamina was. I made it my top priority. I was not going to let cancer define me.

At the tender age of 25, losing my hair had led to a lot of insecurities. I would humor my fiancé by joking about how his hair was longer and more luscious than mine. Despite my insecurities, I am grateful that my fiancé never made me feel any different. I engaged a trainer to help me get started and told her, "We need to go really slow but we'll need to get to the goal." We kickstarted my journey toward fitness and eating well. I would work out a few times a week, and I also had to manage my recovery post each workout. I was happy that we found a routine and my trainer understood my "limitations" but was determined to help me achieve my goals. Despite our efforts, when I stood on the weighing scale, I recall that the number did not change very much. While I could feel myself getting stronger, the number on the scale would leave me frustrated and disheartened.

After the wedding, my husband and I happily settled into a routine. I had begun taking an oral pill every day that managed hormones in my body to keep my cancer in check. I had always been healthy and conscious about my food intake. However, I noticed that after starting the pill, my weight began to increase. Even though there was no medical proof to indicate this, I strongly believed it was a contributing factor. I was exercising and dieting regularly, yet my weight was increasing. I felt so frustrated that I would constantly rant to my husband, "Nothing is working for me! This is so hard!"

In hindsight, I wish I had been more patient with my body. In many ways, I was still in denial about what I had been through. I did not want to accept that my body was different from what it had been before. So, I pushed myself harder by joining a renowned gym that had a reputation for impressive transformations. I later realized that was not the best decision. The training regime set by the fitness trainers did not take into account what my body could handle. The pre-wedding approach of "we need to go really slow, but we'll need to get to the goal" was off the table. In a world where Instagram and other social media constantly remind us what the ideal body is supposed to look like, my efforts often felt like a hopeless pursuit.

"Why don't you try yoga?" a close friend suggested.

I was skeptical because I had always only exercised in a gym. However, I kept an open mind and signed up for the first class. At first, I found most of the yoga poses challenging due to my limited flexibility. I was also wary that my mastectomy and breast reconstruction had reduced muscle mobility. This would lead to tension in the back area, which in turn caused stiffness in my neck and shoulders. But I was determined to keep going. I continued the yoga lessons and soon I even started looking forward to them. Over time, my body was able to do more and more yoga poses and my flexibility improved tremendously.

I also focused on managing my nutrition intake. If one were to attempt to research what diet to follow to prevent the recurrence of cancer, they'd be inundated with information. Cut out processed foods, limit sugar intake, do not eat red meat, limit dairy products, find organic substitutes, and more. The list goes on and on. I followed as much as I could while ensuring that my body was receiving proper nourishment. Even speaking to nutritionists left me more confused because each professional looked down upon the recommendations of the other. I tried out the various diets but nothing seemed to really work. My body would eventually remind me that these solutions were not meant for me. I would have bouts of gastric issues and indigestion. I eventually realized simplicity worked the best for me. My chosen solution—eat all food groups in moderation. After all, life is short, so why shouldn't we enjoy the foods we love. I learned to balance my food intake with brisk walks, light gym exercises, and yoga.

Four and a half years later, I had my relapse and I was back on the chemo chair. I watched as the nurse administered the steroid intravenously. Sigh. I had just found a good rhythm to my fitness routine and diet yet here I was undergoing treatment to save my life, yet again. I felt as though things were out of my control. Fitness was the least of my concerns. Singapore had just gone into a state of lockdown due to the COVID-19 pandemic I was in the hospital every week for my treatment. The pandemic along with the diagnosis of metastatic breast cancer began to make me feel like the world was coming to an end. I turned to food as a coping mechanism during these tough times.

"I have brought you chicken rice," my husband would say when he got food for me during my chemotherapy. Lunchtime always fell in between the sessions. My husband and I would always have chicken rice from the hospital food center. While a part of me knew it was not the healthiest option, the comfort it brought me during my treatment far surpassed the desire to limit myself to a bland meal. I had made it a practice to keep myself happy with treats that I enjoyed. I tried hard to eat healthy during chemo and while most of the time I did, there were times I did not hold back from indulging. I viewed good food as a reward for completing each treatment session. Instead of letting the side effects of the treatment weigh me down, I made food my source of happiness. It helped me to get through the emotional ups and downs the day brought.

My chemotherapy lasted for nine months. At the end of it, I had gained 15 kilos. Maybe it was water retention from the many bags of medication, the comfort eating, the steroids, or everything combined together. I was so grateful to have finished chemotherapy but at the same time, I knew I needed to do something about my fitness, just to feel healthy and strong again. "I am going to go back to the gym for training," I told my husband, feeling good about my decision. I remember I bought a new pair of training shoes that day, wore my new gym clothes, and kickstarted this new routine. However, I eventually realized I could not keep up with the activity, and very often I would fall ill due to over-exhaustion and low energy. I was extremely confused about what to do. My clothes were no longer fitting me well. I dreaded the idea of dressing up as I would have to retry multiple outfits before I felt comfortable in one. I did not feel like socializing as I felt very self-conscious.

"Oh my god, is this even me?" I asked my husband as I saw my reflection in the mirror. It seemed trivial to be upset and obsess over my weight after going through metastatic breast cancer, but my fitness mattered to me. I had lost a part of my identity, my confidence, and self-esteem in my battle against this disease.

This stage was a turning point for me. The weight gain also brought with it the weight of words. People whom I met or interacted with were blatantly hurtful in their feedback and comments, intentional or not I can never be sure.

"Nikita, your face looks swollen."

"Your face is bloated."

"Nikita, are you expecting?"

"Wow! Haven't seen you in so long, how come you gained so much weight?"

"I have a diet plan that worked for me, do you want to know more?"

Even though all of it probably came from a lack of awareness or ignorance, the weight of these words fell on me. They were hurtful to hear. It was truly a rude awakening of how people perceive that weight can be controlled easily and how pervasive the weight stigma can be. After all, in our world parents frequently urge children to lose weight. Social media never fails to feed all the weight-obsession topics such as "What-I-Eat-In-A-Day" YouTube videos, before vs after transformations, and tips and guidelines of dieting. It's a constant reminder of what is the ideal. Though meant to inspire or educate, it inevitably causes people to measure themselves against others.

"Why does it always have to be about appearance? What about the fact that I have just completed my treatment? Why can't people be more sensitive?" I would ask my husband. "There ought to be more empathy in this world."

The first time I got diagnosed I did not fully embrace the lessons that were in front of me. I just wanted to put it all behind me and move on with my life and start my marriage. But when the relapse happened, I stopped and reflected to ask what can I learn from this experience.

During a session with my therapist one day, I was asked, "Have you ever loved your body?" I thought long and hard. There was always so much pressure to look a certain way that I never actually thought positively about my body. Growing up, I was constantly harsh on myself. But now something had changed. I had a new-found respect for my body. It has been there for me; it has endured all the chemotherapy and other medications I had to take; it still supported me every step of the way. So, why was I putting so much pressure on myself? Why was I comparing myself with anyone? In order to make peace and love my body, I had to get rid of the pressure and stop the negativity that weighed on me mentally. The most important realization was that I am enough just the way I am. My body has been beautiful in all the stages of my life and that I am worthy of receiving love and loving myself.

The journey towards self-acceptance has been a challenging one. Discrimination remains rampant but now I choose how I want to react and respond. I believe in emphasizing self-care and encouraging empathy. I remain hopeful that the world we live in will become more empathetic towards fostering respect and understanding and eliminating the stigma of weight gain. The weight of words is far heavier than anyone can imagine.

In conclusion, I am proud of my body and will never let anyone make me feel ashamed of it. Not anymore. I still exercise regularly, and I enjoy swimming and long walks. I am no longer paying attention to restrictive eating regimes or aggressive exercise plans. I thank my body, and I only want to send it love because I understand now what I did not before. I am happier, and I live each day with this motto on my mind, "Be Kind to Yourself."

—Nikita Wadhwani

THE "PHYSICS" OF CANCER

Cancer is very much a mind game. But it is also an intense contact sport. However, before I get started on the physical dimension of cancer, it is probably worth mentioning how utterly unprepared I was for what my body would go through over a six-month period. Growing up, I was not the sporting kind, so there wasn't even a history of broken bones. I had my share of exotic diseases in the past—double vision and facial paralysis—as well as a fair share of infections and fevers, but nothing that really left me miserable and in pain for more than a week.

Strangely, the closest experience, at least from my perspective, was my lifelong battle with chronic acne. And while that feels like comparing the trivial with the torrid, dealing with severe acne through some of the most physically conscious years of my life gave me some unwanted experiences in dealing with body image issues. But that is also somewhat like saying I can fly a plane because I understand the physics of flight. However, in a completely confounding paradox, the month before my cancer diagnosis was also when, at least from a pure measurement standpoint, I was at my fittest.

A childhood of mostly avoiding sport led to a more focused desire to get fitter as the years went by. After several false starts at the gym during my early 20s and a 20 kg body mass accumulation within four years of finishing college, I discovered that running was the first sustained physical activity I enjoyed. The onset of my early 30s and finding a willing partner in my wife, Divya, led to participation in annual half marathons complemented by some gym-based cardio sessions. On occasion, I flirted with yoga. And then, finally, a few years before cancer, I discovered true love in strength training through a phenomenal physical instructor at a gym in Singapore.

That is how I found myself a month before the cancer diagnosis—overweight but not obese, the strongest I had ever been in my life. I had also just completed my best "one-rep max," which is strength training code for bench marking the highest weights one can lift with one repetition. Ironically, it was an intense upper body workout over a weekend that led me to run my hands over the sore parts of my body and discover the lump near my collar bone.

When Mass Becomes Weight

In the three-week window between discovering the lump and starting chemo, I had many difficult experiences. But one experience was singularly strange. That was trying to reconcile what felt like a normal healthy body with the knowledge that it now carried a possibly expanding mortal threat. The surgery I needed to have for biopsy was the closest I had come to experiencing the "ambience" of being sick. The day before chemo I went to the barber intending to shave off my hair. The barber struggled with my sudden news and didn't want to go that far—so I ended up getting a "more than the usual" cut with a "style line" on one side—something I would have never done in regular life. Then there was day one of chemo. My memories of that day are vivid. I went through what eventually would become my "pre-game" ritual. A tried and tested breakfast, plenty of fluids, a prayer session on the phone with a dear friend, and a T-shirt from my gym that said "PHUC Cancer."

The chemo session itself was mostly anticlimactic but with a decent bit of drama. I am terrified of needles. The first failed attempt at finding a vein on my forearm to set up the intravenous chemo treatment sent me into a state of panic. Then there was the tension I could feel at the way the nurses were observing whether

I was having an allergic reaction to any of my four chemo medications. There was also the sudden panic I felt as the steroids I got created a tingle in my body. There was the burning I felt in my veins as they found the right "speed" for the drip. But mostly, I felt drowsy as the anti-allergic medicines took effect. I remember going home and wondering what the big deal about chemo was and that maybe my "fit" body would respond magnificently and with minimal side effects. The next three days were relatively normal. I was taking enough medicines every day to suppress multiple side-effects and while there were no crazy ones, I wasn't feeling the greatest either. And then came the tipping point on day five.

The Theory of Chaos

On day five, I woke up feeling like I had been hit with a sledgehammer. The fatigue was unlike anything I had ever felt before in my life, and I found it hard to just get out of bed and walk. There was no terrible pain, but I remember thinking that if this was how I was going to feel, it would be humanly impossible to go through another 11 rounds of this. It wasn't until day 10 that I believed I had a shot at getting through this treatment.

But before I get that far, I should probably chronicle days five to nine, the five days of hell I had to endure 12 times over a span of six months. Deep fatigue always prevailed in those days, and as I understood the process better, I could connect that to the period when my blood count and immunity were the lowest because of the chemo drugs destroying the fastest growing cells in my body. But every episode also varied a little—a cramped leg that needed an ER trip and a scan to rule out a blood clot, a persistent cough that needed a trip to a scary-looking isolation ER to rule out COVID-19, acute cystitis (an infection of the bladder or lower urinary tract) that had me walking around in pain for hours in the middle of the night. There was also the paranoid behavior—measuring my temperature zillions of times to make sure it was under 38 degrees Celsius or 100 degrees Fahrenheit to avoid a hospital visit and constantly feeling the lump near my neck and imagining it getting bigger or smaller. There was even comic relief sometimes. Like calling my doctor in utter panic one morning to let him know that I was pooping blood, only to realize later that dinner the previous night included beetroots.

There was the physical transformation into a stranger, someone I simply could not recognize in the mirror. It started with the hair loss. One braces for this much-acknowledged chemo fallout but I must admit that it still hit me hard. In my case, all my white hair fell first giving me temporary hope that was quickly dashed as clumps of black hair also started falling. Then came the weight loss. Within four rounds of chemo, I had lost close to 15 kgs and this was despite having a reasonably healthy appetite and with Divya going the extra mile to make sure I was eating healthy flavorful food. I was slowly starting to disappear inside my clothes. Finally, I lost my eyebrows. It seems trivial in hindsight but losing my eyebrows was the final nail in my appearance coffin. I simply struggled to look at myself in the mirror and in some of my darkest hours I just hated the stranger that was looking back at me. In an absurd turn of fate, after almost two decades of battling acne, my skin was finally clear. But I had just stumbled upon the definitive lesson in perspective.

As I cycled through the 12 rounds of chemo, in some ways, knowing how the 14-day period between rounds worked helped me cope better with the physical side effects. Knowledge, in this case, was power. But towards the last few sessions, it felt like my mind and body had become somewhat disconnected. The mind was reasonably strong, but the body had started to revolt. A trip to the hospital now triggered nausea even in the parking lot. I needed someone to hold down my hand as they attempted to find the vein. I had always panicked at the sight of needles but a few dozen blood draws later, the panic was only getting worse. What is remarkable about cancer is the swiftness of the fall from strength. That fall and the corresponding consequences are ugly and difficult. I have no secret recipe to avoid that journey. At best, in moments of clarity, it offered me perspective on the vanity of appearances and the fragility of the human body. Order. Chaos. Acceptance.

Discovering Momentum

I remember the first time I stumbled into day 10 after the first chemo session. The despair driven by the physical condition of days five to nine slowly gave way to hope and optimism as I found myself regaining some level of physical strength and getting past the fatigue. That's when I discovered what would be my newfound passion over the next six months—walking. We have a small terrace garden at home and what started as a simple way to keep my body moving turned into a physical and spiritual refuge of sorts. The amount of time I could walk in a day became my measure of how much strength I had regained from the latest chemo session. And it came with a view. I caught some spectacular sunsets during my evening walks. I waited eagerly to spot the resident pair of oriental pied hornbills as they flew past the terrace, often with a pit stop at a nearby tree, to roost for the night. I called close friends and family during these walks. I participated in a virtual "steps" competition with colleagues at work—I obsessed about hitting the 10 thousand steps mark on all the "good" days. Walking was how I finally found a way to swing back the physical momentum in my favor. A simple activity that still allowed me to push my limits, low as they were during those times. I also did my best to eat well, and Divya went out of her way to make me modified and safe versions of my favorite foods during the "good" days. An indulgence of biryani, pani puri, or a traditional Kerala festival feast did wonders to how I felt physically.

As we crossed the halfway mark and headed for the difficult home stretch, I re-discovered yoga. It started with a cousin in Singapore who is a yoga teacher offering to walk me through some simple exercises. I tried them and it felt great. Then another cousin, who is also a yoga teacher in India, took it up a level. She had helped folks in similar circumstances before, so she knew exactly how to help me push myself while avoiding injury. For me, this phase marked what I called "resurgence." While walking helped me cope, yoga helped me go beyond just coping and into thinking about thriving. At first, the sessions were scary, and I could not believe that I would be able to sustain them. But under expert guidance and by taking it slow and steady, half stretches became full stretches and simple poses moved into more complex ones. At the end of the six-month journey, my body was at its weakest and my appearance was hard to characterize. No walking or yoga insulated me from that, but I do believe that all the walking and yoga that I did allowed me to finish the journey as strong as I possibly could. Cancer has its own, sometimes unstoppable, momentum. The best I could do was to find ways to create my own counter momentum, one step, one stretch, and one pose at a time.

A State of Equilibrium

The last chemo session was more an exercise in relief than one of overt celebration. I was simply grateful that this phase was behind me and that I could now wear the "survivor" label. I gave myself a full month to recuperate. The time to get through days five to nine one more time and then watch day 15 go by without the clock being reset. And to then experience the next 14 days in a way that I had not experienced for a long time. Every day slowly revealed a new positive symptom. Initially, it was just the absence of some of the more painful symptoms. Then, an increase in energy and appetite levels and an overall feeling of wellness. And then, the first signs of the hair coming back, including those eyebrows!

When I returned to work a month after chemo, my body still wore the scorched battle scars of the journey. I give full credit to my colleagues for not flinching at my changed appearance. I found that I really wasn't as self-conscious about how I looked as I had imagined I would be. If I say that after this experience I have zero issues with appearances and that I proudly display the acne scars that embellish my body, I would be lying. However, what is true is that I am less bothered about physical appearances in general. I have met that stranger in the mirror and while we will never be best friends, we can get past the appearances that distinguished us and focus our attention on what remained unchanged or got stronger. My sons, Shiv and Shyam, aged four and one during this journey, respectively, were my ultimate teachers on the subject of appearances. One morning they woke up to find all the hair missing on their daddy's head, acknowledged that it could be the work of a naughty crow, and simply moved on to more important things. No stranger in the mirror in their world.

About a month and a half after chemo I went back to the gym and to strength training. Day one was not some heroic comeback story. I could barely lift the empty bar and the full extent of how weak I had become and how much muscle I had lost fully hit me. But one session at a time, with a ton of support from my trainer and with Divya egging me on, the weights increased, and the muscles started to return. About six months after my last chemo session, I lifted more weights during my one-rep max than I had before cancer. It wasn't exactly full circle, but there was a sense of triumph and a sense of relief that my body could overcome what it had been through.

I still walk when I can, while enjoying the sunsets. I have been falling behind on yoga, but overall, I strive to lead a healthy lifestyle. The battles of the mind and the body were both hard; what differed was not the intensity of the battle but the degree of control one had in being able to respond. In the end though, the cancer journey, like an accelerated microcosm of life itself, isn't a story of conquest; it may have a chapter on resilience but, at least for me, it is a story of acceptance. Acceptance of all the light and all the darkness and simply finding the grace in it all. The grace to accept simply and fully what I cannot change and only focus on what I can.

—Sachin Rajakrishnan

INTIMACY, FERTILITY, AND PARENTING

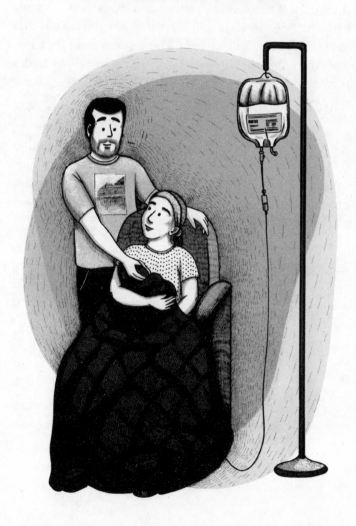

As young adults, cancer robs you of your agency in many ways. It steals your ability to choose who loves you, the way you want to be loved and made love to. The surgery and treatment ravage your body, making you hate the way you look naked in the mirror. When you don't even recognize the person staring back, imagine expecting your partner to love you the way they used to. If you are single, your own insecurities and the taboo around cancer make it almost impossible for you to find a partner.

Many who are starting treatment are often not even informed about its effects on their ability to have children in the future, no matter the gender. Those who are informed or find out themselves and ask for ways to preserve their ability to conceive have to often bear the exorbitant costs of fertility preservation, both financially and physically. So, cancer even nicks your shot at being a parent.

Those who had children pre-diagnosis, got diagnosed during pregnancy, or had preserved their fertility earlier have to face their own distinct challenges. How do you raise a child when you are going through painful treatments? When and what do you tell them about your condition? How do you prepare them when you aren't sure how long you have? Where does this leave your partner? There are no clear answers to any of these questions, but we hope the stories in this section give you some perspective.

MOTHERHOOD INTERRUPTED: LIFE BETWEEN CHEMO AND DIAPERS

When I was young, I used to play house with my friends. We would always role play a lovely close-knit family with a supportive husband, a caring wife, and their cute kids. I would play the wife who would wake up the kids, bathe them, comb their hair, feed everyone healthy food, and then drop the kids at school on the way to her office. It was my happily ever after.

Time flew by. I got married to the love of my life and we moved to Thailand right after. We were both focused on building successful careers, traveling across South-east Asia, and slowly knitting a beautiful life together. It was Christmas eve in 2019 when we were visiting our families in India. My heart must have skipped a beat when the test strip showed "positive." I was pregnant! My husband and I were over the moon! I remember lying in bed together that night, holding hands and thinking about having a baby and our beautiful future together. It was definitely the best Christmas of my life!

I began to make plans about the things I wanted to do during the pregnancy. The Babycenter website had become the most visited place for me on the internet through which I was actively trying to understand the different ways in which my baby was growing in my womb. It was fascinating for me to feel another life developing bit by bit inside me. Even though I had seen my baby only in scans, I had already started to feel like I knew him (I was in Thailand where fetal sex notification is a norm and legal). I knew what kind of music he liked listening to and what kind of gymnastics he was trying in there. I could feel his heartbeat and hoped he could feel mine. I was falling in love with him with every passing day.

The dream of starting this new phase of my life and having my happily ever after was being woven inside my head.

Life, however, had other plans for me. As I was stepping into the 28th week of my pregnancy, I was diagnosed with Classical Hodgkin's Lymphoma—words I had never heard of before. I remember jokingly asking the doctor if this was one of those things that happen during pregnancy and would resolve on its own later. She paused for a bit and then stated that I had cancer.

I didn't know how to respond. At times, it felt so unfair to find myself facing cancer, when all I wanted to think about was the upcoming birth of our child. Instead of giving into the whys and the what ifs, I remember forcing myself to think about my baby. Perhaps, I wanted to divert all my focus on becoming the mother that I always wanted to be and keep the thought of cancer at bay.

The next four weeks were spent in deciding whether or not to have a premature delivery. There was a tussle for the number of days I could let the baby develop inside my womb without risking our lives. We didn't know how fast the cancer was spreading; we didn't know how far it had reached already. And we couldn't find out anything without passing radioactive materials (which were harmful for my fetus) through my body as a part of the PET scan. That meant we had to take my baby out. It was ironic that my body was no longer the safe space where I could nurture this new life.

I remember gently holding my belly and talking to my baby about the fault in our stars. I remember telling him how much I loved him and saying sorry a million times for not being able to protect him inside my womb for as long as I wanted to.

I spent hours talking to pediatricians and hematologists to understand how I could accelerate the growth of my baby and what would be the optimal time to go for a C-section that would give him the highest chances of survival. I found myself advocating for his life even if that meant more risks for me. I delivered my son six weeks before he was ready for this world, and I had to keep him away from me, in the Neonatal Intensive Care Unit (NICU), till he was strong enough. The next few weeks passed in a blur.

When I got discharged from the hospital, I remember feeling the chills of loneliness as I entered an empty house that lacked the celebration of a new birth. All I heard was an eerie silence that seemed to mourn the loss of dreams, the loss of the kind of motherhood I had imagined. I remember that the first thing I did as soon as I got home was to make *halwa* (an Indian sweet) to celebrate the birth of my son, in the hope that I would forget the grief I felt. I visited my baby in the cold NICU multiple times a day, hoping that he would feel the same warmth, the same connection that I did.

Becoming a mother has been an extremely emotional journey for me, full of roller-coaster rides and struggles. Perhaps, the challenges I faced as a new mom weren't unique. But cancer just made them exponentially harder. Motherhood wasn't looking the way I had dreamt it would.

I had planned to spend my maternity leave bonding with my baby, feeding him, playing with him, and exploring the world through a mother's eyes. When I returned to work after, I wanted to still find the time to be the best mother to my son, while having a successful career.

In reality, I was juggling hospital visits, nanny interviews, and looking after my baby with the limited energy I had left. I would spend whole days in the hospital for chemotherapy or related side effects. Then, I would spend my nights dealing with sleeplessness from the pains. When I would be awake at night, I would often look at my baby. Many times, he would smile in his sleep and it would give me peace. My online reading shifted between my symptoms and baby milestones. I was learning to inject blood thinners into my body while also learning to set up a night routine for my baby. I had not one but two demanding new jobs (cancer patient and a new mother) to manage. I was not (just) a mother, I had become a mother with cancer.

Being a mother with cancer meant less energy and time, plus a ton of limitations. I remember when my premature baby was born, he was struggling to digest formula milk. His weight wasn't increasing and the doctors at the NICU were worried. Breast milk feeds were a solution, but I only had a week to provide as much as I possibly could. I had my PET scan in a week and after that my milk would have become toxic for my own baby. I took to breast pumping like crazy. I did as much as I could to support his health and be as much of a mother as I could be. The breast milk worked and slowly his stomach matured. He adapted to formula milk but became colic and had a series of constipated days for the first few months. We consulted many doctors and every time I had to explain why I wasn't able to provide my breastmilk I felt helpless. I remember how hurt I was when someone made an offer to my husband to provide their breastmilk to support my baby. It just made me feel so much less as a mother at the time. In hindsight, accepting the offer was better than seeing him suffer from colic.

When I had thought of having a child, nobody had prepared me for the tremendous amount of effort, commitment, and energy it takes to raise one. Perhaps, like most people from India, I was relying on having our parents around to guide us through parenting. And well, nobody prepares you to have cancer. Both the new roles I had demanded a lot of energy and needed a lot of support. On both fronts, I found myself lacking.

Even the timing didn't work in our favor. Due to COVID-19 restrictions our parents couldn't be around. I must have called, emailed, and begged so many people at the embassy to somehow get my parents to support us in Thailand. While they were sympathetic, they couldn't do anything. All they could offer was to transport us to India instead. However, at the time COVID-19 was spreading like wildfire in India. It just didn't make sense to put myself and my baby at risk by traveling there. My only option was to build my support system in Thailand.

While we wanted to hire help, finding a reliable nanny was not easy. Especially since I was looking for someone who could literally replace me when I was not around. Most nannies I interviewed were used to being the helper while the mother took care of the baby. I remember spending the first few minutes in every interview explaining my limitations to the candidate and how it added to their responsibilities. Many candidates we liked didn't show up because they found another job that required them to do a lot less. I finally hired a nanny who would stay eight hours in the day while I took care of all the night duties. It seemed doable when we started out as I still felt okay health-wise. That said, I was miserable on many days. I remember my baby would have bouts of colic just around the time my nanny left and there was unstoppable crying for hours at a stretch. I would hold him, rock him, walk him, constantly telling him how much I loved him. Sometimes, we would both cry.

It was difficult for me to accept my low energy levels and my own limitations as a mother. Many times, it felt like I was doing my best yet failing to keep up. My husband was the only family I had around. But he kept busy. Busier than I had hoped. While he would listen to my repetitive complaints about pain and sometimes applied balm on my aching feet at night, he couldn't find the time to go to many of my follow ups and not a single one of my radiations. Though he would spend time with our son after work and many times we took turns rocking him to provide relief from colic, his work was always the priority and it made me feel less important and less supported. Perhaps, he was also coping with the additional responsibilities at work and the new role he now had. But it all made me feel lonely. The time I spent with my son was the only solace I had.

Soon my body stopped cooperating with the mother in me. I started having peripheral neuropathy and veinal thrombosis. My arms had massive swelling and pain. Every day, I would apply balm and tie crepe bandages around them and inject blood thinners in my body along with strong painkillers. I would often cry through the nights as it became difficult for me to hold my baby and rock him to sleep. I felt like a failure. I needed help and I didn't know where to find it.

I posted on my local mummies' Facebook group to find alternatives for help during the night. Someone told us to seek the help of Thai nannies who stayed with the baby 24 hours and took care of everything. After much struggle, we found such a nanny. She didn't know English but we managed to talk to each other through Google Translate. It was surely difficult but it was better than having no help at all.

My health was deteriorating with every chemo cycle, and I was no longer available for baby care. The nanny was taking care of him completely. There were days I would feel happy to have found the support system I needed. On other days I would feel sad. My son wouldn't show the same affection to me as he would show toward her. I didn't feel like his mother.

She stuck around for one and a half months before going back to her hometown to take care of some family matters. Her departure meant I was back to square one, making trade-offs like avoiding drowsy medicines to be more alert for baby care. I felt cranky, and I hoped it was out of sleep deprivation rather than a lack of love for my baby. "Am I a bad mother?" I often thought.

Despite my efforts, my little baby of three and a half months was silent for two days. It was almost as if he was grieving the separation from his beloved nanny. It was devastating for me to see my baby suffer and yet not be able to do much. It made me feel completely helpless and powerless.

After that incident, I decided to be the constant in his life, no matter how many nannies we changed. I hired extra help and outsourced all other things, except my medical stuff. I also started to stack up my appointments, optimizing my hospital days like a ninja. I would come up with creative ways to bond with him despite my limitations. It was as if I had found my spark in becoming the mother for him who was his constant. I am not sure if I would have gone that extra mile if life would have been smoother for me. My misery pushed me to create that special bond I have with my son in which we are independent yet full of love. This will always be my silver lining!

During my pregnancy I always imagined myself wearing a suit, carrying my baby in a stroller, walking around with a laptop, and being the woman who had it all worked out. But then cancer happened. With the kind of support (or the lack of it) I had, at the three-month mark, when my maternity leave was coming to an end, I clearly couldn't return to work. I was in too much pain physically, too exhausted mentally, and was still struggling to find a permanent support system at home. Work took a backseat.

My employer was supportive and we agreed on a three-month extension. Those three-months also passed in a blink of an eye. I had finished eight sessions of chemotherapy and 20 radiation sessions; I still hadn't found reliable help for baby care. When the time came to get back to full-time work, I was hesitant. With support from my organization, I decided to start with part-time work hours for a month and set up my own pace. Month after month I kept on seeking extensions. In the beginning, it was primarily to support my own health, but eventually, it was just the lack of support. Every time a nanny left, all baby care responsibilities would fall on me. My husband still wasn't ready to equally share the baby duties. So, I would need to take time off work, take care of the baby, and conduct nanny interviews. If we got lucky in finding a nanny, I had to train them all over again. At times it felt like my career wasn't as important. I was clearly far away from my dream of "I-can-have-it-all." The lack of support made me angry.

Whenever I would discuss my situation with my family and friends, they kept giving me their opinions on whether or not I should continue working. I knew I would be unhappy if I didn't have financial independence and let myself get absorbed into baby care 24/7, but I couldn't get back unless I had a stable support system. I struggled with this for quite some time. But the more I thought about it, the more I wanted to surrender. No matter how much it angered me, I decided to pull myself out of the career race (at least for a while), continue my part-time work, take care of my son, and accelerate my career when the time came.

I often reflect on how different my motherhood story has turned out to be and how much has happened in the last two years. The fear of passing cancer on to my son lurks constantly in my mind. It is something I cannot control and have no option but to make peace with. I'm not sure if I am the best mother to my son or what the future holds for us, but I do know that what we went through together will always hold a special place in my heart. That is perhaps the bond that we will always share.

—Thanisha Sehgal

I AM NOT THE FIRST

More than I, if truth were told,
Have stood and sweated hot and cold,
And through their reins in ice and fire
Fear contended with desire.

—*A. E. Housman*

Let alone desires of the body and the mind, expressing desires of any kind is a taboo in our society and is still frowned upon. I do not necessarily mean to talk about sex. Even demanding subtle intimacy and everyday romance can make you feel embarrassed and judged.

How can you even think about being a romantic when you are struggling with a life-threatening disease? I often asked myself. Just like everyone else, I too was accustomed to thinking that love and romance were not meant for someone who has a long-term illness and that too a dreaded disease like cancer. I was diagnosed with breast cancer in December 2019, at the age of 31. As a young girl, I used to consider myself beautiful. If not as popular, in the literal sense of the word, I had my fair share of admirers, including myself.

Cancer robs you of the agency over your own body in more ways than one. Even though it had not spread in my body, the doctors suggested that I should go for chemotherapy because of a strong family history of breast and ovarian cancer in my paternal lineage. I was scared to undergo the genetic testing to find out if I had a genetic mutation that would increase the possibility of me facing the same fate as others before me. I feared it would be positive. Despite my doctor's insistence, I refused to take the test though I was prepared to undergo the prescribed treatment. She suggested that I could either undergo mastectomy (removing the affected breast completely) or conserve some part of my right breast (where the malignant lump resided) by opting for lumpectomy with sentinel lymph node biopsy. Selecting the second method meant that only the breast tissues around the suspicious site would be removed and not the breast altogether. This sounded better and somehow easier to me. At least I would be able to retain some semblance of my old self if not entirely. I thought, what is a woman without her breasts? Is she still a woman? I didn't know and still don't have an answer for it. Such thoughts aside, my treatment came with a condition that post surgery and chemotherapy I would be subjected to radiotherapy. I didn't realize what I had signed up for and the toll it would take on my body; however, reluctantly I accepted it.

The course of breast surgery, chemotherapy, and radiotherapy not only impacted my body from the inside but also made me look like a ghost version of myself on the outside. The scars on my body were too many to count. They took a lot of time to heal and made me self-conscious of my body. Chemotherapy made it worse. I had my hair cut very short even before it started, anticipating the hair loss, thinking that their short length would make me suffer less. That didn't help. It was still very painful to lose them strand by strand. My skin and nails started darkening, and I started losing even my eye brows and eye lashes. My eyes began to lose their sparkle. While on one hand I was struggling to even look at myself in the mirror, on the other, I still wanted my partner to display expressions of love and care for me.

That did not happen. He ignored my constant requests by calling them complaints. He believed that I was victimizing myself and that my demands were futile. My heart bled. I had several sleepless nights. I couldn't stop blaming myself for my fate. I started measuring my worth based on my new appearance.

The sense of aloofness did not start with my disease. Even when I was young, I struggled to speak my heart out. Suppressing my feelings came naturally to me. And when I faced my most difficult battle with this disease, a subtle metamorphosis seemed to have begun. I wanted to be more authentic in my display of opinion on any matter. I wanted to clearly state what I wanted out of my life. I learned it the hard way that no matter how good or difficult the situation is, we, and only we are responsible for our happiness or misery. And if I am unable to do anything, I am the only one to be blamed. I was slowly becoming more self-aware and self-centered, in every sense of the word.

All through my treatment, even with my friends and family around, I felt lonely and desolate. When I tried to discuss romance and love while having a catheter attached to my veins, it didn't go down well with them. No one really understood. I think they didn't realize that more than ever, now was the time I was seeking solace in my near and dear ones. All I was looking for was a shoulder to lean on, an eager ear to hear me out and care about what I had to say, a gentle touch, and a loving glance to reassure me that I was still beautiful and desired. When I demanded it, I was silenced, time and time again. People generally believe that one's fears and emptiness should not be discussed so openly. On top of that, how can we talk about intimate issues blatantly, especially as women? After all, aren't we always taught: "Girls shouldn't talk like that!"

Intimacy, both physical and emotional, is important to foster any relationship. And more so for a cancer patient with a deformed body who is anxious about the future and their health and has hormonal imbalances that sometimes make it difficult to even feel an emotion completely. Oddly, all these feelings somehow led to a lot of extremes such as easy irritability, absolute emptiness, bouts of fear, unreasonable urges to laugh out loud, and even a reduced urge to go through the physical act of making love.

But that does not diminish the need to feel loved and longed for. When my desire for hugs was returned with half-hearted gestures or my need to hold hands was so carelessly ignored, it made a deep dent in my soul. If only the partners and caregivers could understand the vulnerabilities of cancer patients and survivors. Come to think of it, if one feels loved and important, it increases their will to live on. And that is the best medicine to improve their health. In my case, however, I was struggling to keep myself afloat.

There is a constant battle in your head about whether you should reveal your disfigurement and scars to the world while putting up a brave smiling face. I was uncomfortable with my situation but was trying to accept it. Caught in this dichotomy of my circumstances, I realized that the journey through this treatment would be imperfect, just like life is. When it all started, I was clueless, vulnerable, and completely shattered. I was losing and gathering some parts of myself each day. When COVID-19 hit, my situation worsened. I was unable to see anyone except for my partner for a long time. As the circles of support became smaller and smaller, I gradually began to accept my situation and change my life with each passing day.

Chemo Can Make You Infertile. Really?

Since I was diagnosed with cancer at a young age, I had not reached the stage of family planning. The blow of going through chemotherapy was huge! From all that I got to learn, it was supposed to be a toxic therapy that kills good cells in the body along with the malignant ones. It impacts hair follicles, skin, nails, and even the digestive system. Later, a thorough discussion with my doctor made me realize that it could hugely impact my fertility and chances of becoming a mother as well.

Thankfully, while sharing this heart breaking news, she also gave me a way out. She introduced us to oocyte cryopreservation, wherein eggs harvested from my ovaries surgically would be preserved for later use. This technique greatly increased our chances of bearing a child in the future, if we decided to have one.

Surprisingly, it wasn't as difficult to have a discussion about this procedure with my family. Not as tough as I had anticipated. Although it was a tough call, my situation demanded us to make a quick decision.

Right from the second day of my surgery in which I went through lumpectomy (partial removal of breast tissue) and sentinel lymph node biopsy, I took hormonal injections to stimulate ova production in the body. The injections were not only painful but also caused a lot of uneasiness. The physical pain and the mental disquiet were overwhelming. I had so many needles poking my stomach and my back that I couldn't even think straight. Moreover, the discomfort of an uncertain future was playing havoc with my mind and body. While I was feeling confident about my decision, there was still grief and pain. Nevertheless, I went with the flow.

When I look back at those ten days now, I feel proud of myself for making a smart decision. It gives me immense joy and confidence because I know that I am giving myself a chance to bounce back and have a child in the future, if and when I feel ready for it.

Boundaries and Difficult Conversations

I believe that no one should have to justify their thoughts or life choices unless they are physically harmful or traumatizing for other people. Sometimes we just forget to create boundaries around ourselves, especially with respect to difficult conversations such as choosing to be a mother or claiming our sexuality.

In a conversation with a fellow patient, I learned that she was not allowed to remove her breasts just to keep looking like a "woman." Her cancer relapsed with metastases, and later, she succumbed to it. The price we pay to look and feel like "women" is agonizing to say the least. In another discussion with my doctor, the case of a patient who was not allowed to opt for oocyte cryopreservation came up. The reason the family gave was "that has never happened in our family." As patients, we are often not allowed to take charge of our own bodies and we suffer as a result of the decisions made by others. I believe all patients should have the agency to decide the course of their treatment. When we give the reins of our lives to someone else, we live with regret and angst forever. I, like most others, had my fair share of struggles and learned the lesson the hard way. All that I have understood is that we need to claim our choices ferociously and unabashedly.

I remember feeling agitated by everyday conversations around me during my treatment. It didn't help that my near and dear ones blamed my fate or past life karma for the disease I developed. Nor did it help that people came to me with their toxic positivity quotes. All I expected was a calm environment around me and a regular life. Was it too much to ask for?

I believe it is all right to feel dejected at times and share your feelings with those around you. Living through a life-changing disease is a constant struggle. If there are days you feel angry and sad, accept it as a part of your coping process. Don't run away from your truth.

I Am Not Trying to Give a Pep Talk Here...

In the two years that I have lived with cancer, I have found the courage to get the genetic testing done. I had to learn to accept the fact that I am in fact a BRCA 1 gene mutation carrier and that is why I had to face a cancerous development at a young age. Since I had a very rare type of invasive papillary carcinoma, which is aggressive in nature, I was subjected to a harsh treatment.

I recently completed my prophylactic bilateral mastectomy (complete removal of both the breasts) with cosmetic reconstruction. I move around confidently with only one breast (the other one is still under construction). Mastectomy was a difficult but necessary decision due to medical reasons. It greatly reduces the chances of a recurrence.

I had the consent of my family for this surgery, but I completely owned the decision.

It felt good, until the day before the surgery! The day of my surgery and some days after it were very hard. I felt weak, vulnerable, and unsure again. I came back home with remorse once the procedure had been completed. I was in a lot of pain and this time with no family or friends around I felt even more dejected. The physical scars healed within three weeks, but my thoughts are still a work in progress. I think I am bouncing back, slowly and gently.

The "cancer journey" is bumpy, and it is okay to ride through it the way you feel is right. Some days, I struggle with my body image but on others, I feel motivated to take care of myself to regenerate my inner beauty and youth. I dress up and put on make-up. I accept the desires of my physical body and that of my mind. I count the small wins when I can indulge in self-appreciation and confide in people I trust. My best friend says that I have never looked better in life!

—Vani Verma

NAVIGATING COLLEGE AND CAREER

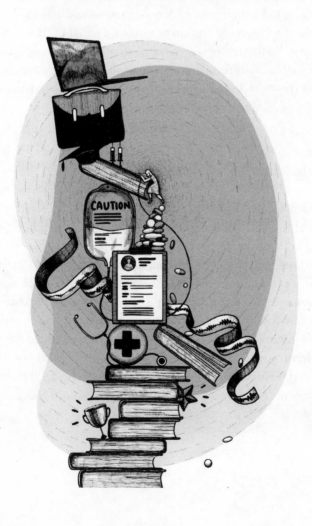

Young adults in the age group of 17 to 39 are usually in their most productive years. Starting and graduating from college, joining and growing at work, and beginning or completing higher education all happen in this period. Imagine racing to the top on a thin dirt road along the edge of a mountain, so close to the peak as a student or professional and suddenly being thrown in the air due to a massive speed breaker called cancer. You're trying very hard to steer yourself from falling off the path to certain death. Your life has come to a standstill after this near-death experience. You gather yourself, breathe, and feel grateful to be alive.

You go into treatment and push through it all. If you are fortunate enough to have been cured or are well enough, you get back to college or work in some form or shape. A few of you might return to your previous careers that you were passionate about, albeit with an acute awareness of the fragility of your life. You might make sure you give your home, hobbies, and health as much time and energy, if not more, than work. At times, you may also have an existential crisis that makes you re-evaluate your entire life, including your career choices. You might decide to do something else altogether or change the way you work completely. From working in one industry to switching to something different you always wanted to try, or from working full-time to a portfolio career with different gigs. Here are some stories of co-authors from very different phases of their careers who found their own way through this maze.

PILOTING MY CAREER THROUGH THE CANCER STORM

Before I get into discussing how cancer crisscrossed my career, I cannot help but reflect on the fact that my current career trajectory owes its beginnings to a health issue. Back in 2003, in my final year at engineering college, I was elated when I landed my first job at one of the Indian software majors through campus placement. That career ended even before it began, as in the last month of college, I found myself with a rescinded offer letter because I had failed the color blindness segment of the medical test. Most of the companies had finished their placement season by then. My worst nightmare had come true.

The standard middle-class upbringing in India prepares you to get to this one moment, when, through your laser-sharp focus on education, you land that one job that provides stability for the rest of your life. That moment had literally slipped right out of my hands. Then, as if it was meant to happen, an MNC showed up—I was the only one from my college who was offered a role at this company during the very last week of college. I have been working for the same company for 19+ years—apparently a statistical outlier in these times. One would think that this early experience was preparation for a more serious health challenge that would come 18 years later.

The truth is that while that experience was an early lesson in resilience, it also left me with a deep-rooted fear of how a health issue can abruptly end one's career. To this day, I remember the nervousness with which I went through the medical test required by my new company when I joined them. One of life's mysteries is that I was not classified as color blind this time, not that my new company seemed to care. Then, within the first six months of joining, I came down with chicken pox and I remember the same nervousness came back to haunt me when I had to miss two weeks of work. Once again, everyone seemed okay with it and life went on.

After that initial phase, I never really encountered any significant health challenges as I navigated through my career—moving across functions, countries, and business segments. In 2010, I landed at the division that was a dream come true—the aviation business. What is not to love about jet engines? People often asked me why I stayed this long at one company. My answer has always been that I loved what I did, loved the product and loved the colleagues I worked with. I had seen colleagues go through health challenges, and I had seen them receive support from the organization and their co-workers. However, I had never given that aspect any deep thought. Throughout my entire career, I had never taken more than two weeks off at a time for any reason. I had the stability that came from being in one company for so long, but even with all that I was simply not prepared for the mid-air collision that was about to unfold when cancer met my career.

Pre-flight Checklist

My diagnosis was sudden. We had wrapped up the 2020 holiday season feeling great as a family. COVID-19 seemed behind us. Divya and I had welcomed our second son into our lives, and at work, I had wrapped up my first year in one of my all-time favorite roles that I had been promoted to at the beginning of the year. We were on a high. Then in Jan 2021, within a span of two weeks, all of it unraveled.

What seemed like a muscle catch from working out at the gym, quickly progressed through various tests over two weeks and ended with a diagnosis of Stage 4 lymphoma. I think the truth is that I did not even fully register what was going on. The medical appointments keep you busy but deep down the mind is in denial. I know, for many, the big question after the diagnosis is with whom and how many should the news be shared.

Looking back, I don't think I spent too much time pondering over this question or even deeply considering the consequences of my choice. Initially, I kept my manager and team in the loop as I was going through the diagnosis process. Then, I automatically told them the final diagnosis without thinking much. I recall being asked if I was comfortable with the news being shared more broadly. I remember discussing it with Divya and reflecting on a general principle I had from my childhood that lies were too much work to manage and maintain. I followed the same principle for cancer— I would tell the truth, but I would make no effort to announce my condition to the world, even as I had no issues with the world knowing about it. I let close colleagues, my team, and folks I worked with on a day-to-day basis learn about my condition and also made it clear that I had no desire to keep this a secret, which allowed folks to talk to each other about it.

From my perspective, letting people know was not an act of bravery because my deepest fear at work was not people knowing about my condition. Having seen close friends and family battle cancer, I carried no stigma in my head about being a cancer patient myself. My deepest fear, I would discover, had not changed much from 2003. It was the fear of losing my job and the stakes seemed higher this time with two little kids in the mix and the risk of losing a career I had built over time.

It would be nice to say that my initial willingness to be open was to inspire others, but it was far from that. It was simply me going through a checklist and making a decision that seemed practical at that time. As I look back at that decision with the clarity and wisdom of hindsight, I am glad I chose that path. In the beginning, it allowed colleagues and friends to feel comfortable about reaching out to me. My detailed response to an email or text would then lead to a more detailed exchange or a conversation. I received help, support, and plenty of great advice. Some of it was tactical, like connecting me to my company's regional medical head who acted as an extra sounding board for my diagnosis and treatment plan. There were a lot of offers of support. A particular email that stood out was from a colleague whose daughter had gone through a similar battle. It shared advice from a caregiver's perspective; advice that kept me grounded about what Divya was likely going through and kept me from adding to her burden mentally. I would have been deprived of this perspective if I had not chosen to be open about what I was going through. Others opened up about what they were experiencing in their lives and those conversations eventually allowed me to see past my own troubles and set the foundation for a deeper empathy when I returned to work. Over time being open also enabled me to receive help from colleagues, help we needed and learned to welcome.

Letting Go During Turbulence

I hit turbulence almost immediately. It seems silly now, but my deepest fear, at least in those early days, was not of dying. Despite being locked in a fight with a disease that could kill me and despite working at a company for 18+ years, what I listed as my top fear in a mail to a colleague was somewhat counterintuitive:

"How do I keep working through chemo... I think my real fear is that if I took six months away from work, I would simply become irrelevant."

A part of me knew that my fear was somewhat illogical. But it was hard to shake off the fear of becoming irrelevant at work. Of not having a job. Of not having the health care benefits and the financial stability that came with the job. I had not had a single conversation at work that hinted that any of these fears would come true, but they would not go away so easily. When my manager asked me to come up with a six-month transition plan, my first version was a mild transition at best. I simply could not imagine being away from work for six months when I had no idea what chemo might feel like. I relied on an optimistic interpretation and imagined that except for a few days I could work normally. COVID-19 had already normalized working from home to my advantage. I just struggled to let go, partly because I felt accountable but mostly because I was terrified to let go.

There was no easy way to create a better transition plan, but I received help. When I asked my oncologist if I could keep up with my regular work responsibilities while going through treatment, I really hoped he would reassure me. But he was brutally honest and told me that while I could do whatever I was capable of during chemo, his only priority and focus was to help me beat cancer with an effective treatment plan and that I ought to change my mindset to focus on that as well. It was a tough pill to swallow. I remember walking out of his clinic feeling somewhat lost, but that conversation eventually helped me shake out of my badly prioritized battle order.

My manager, who by then had done his homework on side effects of chemo, insisted on a revised transition plan that required me to own nothing for six months but gave me the flexibility to participate in whatever I could. The organization clearly offered unequivocal support—take the time you need to overcome this and come back when you are ready. While it didn't completely kill the fear, it helped take the edge off. And finally, for inspiration, I took to heart advice from an ex-US Airforce pilot's talk at work where she suggested that when flying in formation, the natural tendency during turbulence is to hold the controls harder but what helps is loosening the grip and going with the flow. I imagined myself doing that.

In the end, I created a transition plan that did not have my name on it. I fully delegated my responsibilities to my team. I was immensely lucky to work at an organization that supported me in my time of need. The personal relationships I had built over my long tenure helped me manage my own irrational fears. And some days as I lay in bed wrecked by the side effects of chemo, I was just grateful that I chose to let go and take the time to focus on enduring and healing.

Watching the Planes Fly

Any misgivings about letting go at work quickly disappeared around day five of the first chemo session, and I started getting a better sense of what my body would go through over the 12 prescribed chemo sessions. While the first four days lulled me into a false sense of security, on day five I woke up to find that I literally had no strength to get out of bed. The fatigue was unlike anything I had experienced before. I could not focus on anything. Reading a book or even watching a movie somehow seemed painful. But by day 10, the body started to recover its strength and the mind its focus, and I started getting a sense of the cyclical nature of chemotherapy.

Break. Build. Rinse. Repeat.

Once I understood the pattern of good and bad days, I also started to leverage the flexibility I had at work and selectively participated in work activities and projects that were not time sensitive. I kept my team and manager updated on what I was going through via a series of periodic emails. I pulled back from the day-to-day topics, skipped or remained silent at meetings I joined so as not to cause confusion in the organization, and made myself available as a sounding board when needed.

The first couple of months were hard and sometimes awkward as I struggled to find a balance but over time this became easier. I was able to get past my own fears and insecurities and simply listen. The spectator mode sometimes worked as a distraction from the effects of chemo and at other times allowed me to quietly take pride in how my team was running the show on their own. Again, the way I stayed connected to the organization through my six-month break was not the consequence of a well-planned process. What worked was a few general principles—for starters, knowing the priority of the battle and learning to trust and let go, and later, organically finding ways to stay engaged, partly for selfish reasons but also to contribute and give back for all the help I was receiving, including the extra load my team was taking on to compensate for my absence.

Through this period, I was also the beneficiary of an incredible amount of support from my colleagues. Some folks made sure they always texted or called me around chemo sessions or PET scan milestones. We received flowers, cakes, cards, books, a meditation mat, and gift subscriptions to online classes and apps. Some came in on Sundays to help Divya with the kiddos. My manager sent me a cap representing our favorite sports team which I ritually wore to every chemo session. The office ran a roster system to coordinate hospital drops for blood work or chemo. This gave Divya some breathing space but also allowed me to connect in person with a colleague every other week. On the day of my first scan about two months after chemo had started, a colleague dropped a box with 50+ postcards—handwritten by colleagues from 5+ countries. I think that was the first time I cried since the beginning of the cancer journey. I was deeply moved.

I learned a lot of lessons in this phase. I learned how poor a listener I really had been as I now listened to meetings and finally understood what it meant to listen to understand instead of just listening to respond. I learned about how an empowered team could really step up and work wonders and I was humbled by how my team operated without me. I reflected on how I would empower my team, even more, when I returned. But most importantly as I reflected on how my colleagues' acts of support strengthened and motivated me, I wanted to be a better colleague at work and give back to an organization and to colleagues who had given me so much.

Flying Anew

The initial fears gave way to a more reconciled peace for most of the treatment period, at least in the way I interacted with work and with my colleagues. That steady phase also left me somewhat unprepared for the transition back to work. As I wrapped up chemo and waded through the extra month of healing and recovery, I was gripped with anxiety for a variety of reasons. The fears of losing my job because I was out for six months had now started to actually look silly, but they were quickly being replaced by other fears. I was terrified of a relapse and in addition to not being able to imagine going through the same process all over again, I was now also wondering how the organization would deal with me having to be out for an extended period again. Once again, this was not based on anything rational. I was also worried if my body and mind could cope with the pressures of work again. Worse, I worried whether after the whole process of reflection on life and death, I would feel motivated by a work deadline ever again.

A few things helped with the transition back. The first was finding a way to cope with the fear of relapse. There is no silver bullet to this one. But what I endured allowed me to be more accepting of what I could not control. At some point, you acknowledge all your deepest fears. In my case, I talked to Divya about them, and then I just found a box in the corner of my mind to lock them down. They exist, but mostly, they don't interfere. The other thing that helped me was a deep sense of gratitude. I was grateful for what my work had enabled in my life and how all of that helped me navigate the cancer journey. I was looking forward to finding ways to give back to the organization and my colleagues. Finally, in the quietness of cancer, I had also developed clarity about why I wanted to work, beyond just paying the bills. My days needed purpose and camaraderie, the purpose of working on problems that mattered and the camaraderie of people to solve them with.

I didn't quite expect it, but the first few months of getting back to work were, at least in my head, days when I did some of the best work of my life. I was simply happy to be able to work every day. There wasn't a thing at work that could stress me, and I found that I could compartmentalize and switch on and off at ease between work and play. The quietness of the past few months lingered on and the lack of noise and chatter in the head was exhilarating. I was more candid than I had ever been, and I was more conscious of how I spent my time at work. I also started carrying the torch for more balance between work and life outside of work, determined to remind everyone that we could not put off life until our working careers were over. I truly believed that we could do the best work of our lives while living our best lives.

I wish that this was some form of permanent euphoria. Unfortunately, with time the mind put some layers to distance me from the traumatic events. I have found that it is sometimes hard to remember and hold on to the lessons I learned, to hold on to the clarity that came from six months of quietness. I find myself at times slipping back into the old habits, taking on that meaningless work deliverable, worrying about the next job, working late when I should be playing with the boys, being less empathetic and thoughtful towards a work colleague than I should be, letting the stress creep in, worrying about what others think of me, and much more. But at least until now, I find it easier to recognize that drift. When it happens, I simply remind myself of all that I went through, and I reset. And I fly on.

—Sachin Rajakrishnan

REIMAGINING YOUR LIFE, RECALIBRATING YOUR CAREER

What do you do when you have had a near-death experience and feel like you have been reborn? What do you do when you realize that your potential expiry date may not be too far away? How do you continue doing the boring and mundane things you did in the hopes of a better future, pushing your actual dreams for an imaginary "later" and procrastinating because you felt like you had "a lot of time"? What do you do when life gives you a second chance, a do-over, a clean slate to do things the way you actually wanted to? This is what happened to me when I was diagnosed.

I spiraled into a long existential crisis, a journey that can be caging and releasing at the same time. I felt trapped because I realized that I was never truly living for myself; I did all that others asked me to do, expected of me, and I believed I ought to do. The weight drowned me, instead of helping me float. But the journey can be liberating too because I finally realized I didn't need to do all of that anymore. I am living for myself first and then *if* (and a big IF!) something aligns with my values, dreams, and goals, I'll do things for others as well. My primary responsibility is to myself, whatever that may be. For instance, my non-negotiable value is service to others. I just can't do something which I know will, even if eventually, cause any harm to others. I find meaning and joy in being able to help, support, and enable people to be their best selves. Injustice of any kind riles me up. As an activist at heart, a few causes are very dear to me. I stand up and advocate strongly for them. But I have had to tone it all down for a long time to fit into the expectations that my parents and the world of work had from me. However, I am no longer willing to censor myself. I shall share my story boldly, speak truth to power, and face the music when necessary but continue to fight the good fight. I have one life after all, and a short one at that. I'd like to do things that make a difference and perhaps a tiny dent in the universe while I'm at it.

When faced with death, humans tend to think about how they'd like to be remembered when they are gone. This need to leave a legacy behind in the grand scheme of things, where millions of people take birth and perish every day, is what makes us human. We do it to not be just another statistic, to not be forgotten, to be remembered for posterity, to become immortal in some way. It is a way to escape the finality and nothingness of death, which scares us all. Some try to do it through their inventions, businesses, and philanthropy, others through their love and support for their near and dear ones. Many make amends in their relationships. A few try new things to avoid dying with regrets. Fewer still want to leave bigger legacies behind. I imagine myself to be one of the latter kind. I strive to serve all the communities that I now belong to and make a tangible impact on the lives of those within them—for all those who already belong now and will become, unfortunately with no choice or agency of their own, their part in the future.

Under the weight of all these realizations, how do you continue doing what you did before? How do you not question, challenge, and deconstruct what led you to do what you were doing, what you actually wanted to do with your life, and where you are today? It is but obvious that one reimagines their life and their limited futures and recalibrates their priorities under these circumstances. The process of doing this creates an identity crisis of sorts, one that may lead you to question your entire existence. We have a tendency to identify ourselves mainly with our jobs. You may have noticed, when asked to introduce themselves to a stranger, after sharing their names, people don't say, "I consult companies on how to become more profitable," "I help design meaningful learning experiences," or "I help companies code programs that sift through large amounts of data and derive meaningful insights." They instead say, "I'm a consultant," "I'm a learning designer," or "I'm a data analyst." We make our "doing" our "being", that is, we make our work our identity. So, what do you do when your life has been turned upside down, when perhaps you can't work the same way you used to anymore?

I strongly questioned why I did what I did up until now and then I didn't know if I wanted to continue down the same path anymore. Heck, I questioned everything. Was it all worth the lack of work-life balance, the missed meals, late nights, and working weekends? Not to forget the fad diets and extreme workouts I did to attain the "ideal" body. I'm positive that my lack of attention to physical health and deteriorating mental health in the past few years made things worse for me. I remember having multiple mental breakdowns. The thought of waking up each day to get back to work gave me severe panic attacks when all I heard from work was—you weren't doing enough. You weren't working hard enough, you weren't challenging yourself enough, you weren't ambitious enough, you weren't pushing your team enough. I kept wondering—will I ever be enough because even when I was working myself to my bones it wasn't enough. I would hate myself each day if I didn't feel like I had done enough. And all of this when I was working in a field that I was deeply passionate about.

I still vividly remember how I completely broke down one day in my flatmate's room after wrapping up a particularly long day at work. I just couldn't stop crying. I felt completely worthless. It was then that I finally experienced and understood how capitalism reduces us to our output—in a workplace, we are no longer humans, but resources, just like machines. Our value is based on how much we do and keep doing. Despite the wear and tear, we are expected to always do more than before. I had an epiphany that I was just another cog in the wheel in a giant system that constantly threatened to replace me if I didn't meet its expectations, however unrealistic they might be. Over the years, I was indoctrinated to evaluate my self-worth based on how productive I was, how much others appreciated or respected me, and how well or soon I climbed the career ladder. However, I was getting tired of the rat race. Maybe this worked for others, but it wasn't for me. I was pushed to my limits, and I was just a straw away from taking my own life. So, I sought help and reached out to a therapist, whom I have consulted ever since.

Imagine being so close to death, not once but twice. Clearly, I needed to change both how I evaluated my self-worth and how I worked. I was diagnosed just as I was about to start my master's program at Harvard. So, when my doctors told me that I had to keep my stress levels low at all costs to avoid major seizures and cancer recurrences, in a knee-jerk reaction, I decided I wouldn't go back to Harvard, as it might be stressful to do a master's program. But to avoid regrets later, I got myself a two-year deferral, both to give myself enough time to heal and to think about whether I wanted to finish what I had started. This meant I had no option but to go back to the drawing board to figure out what I would do professionally. I certainly didn't want to just sit at home and do nothing, but I couldn't go back to business as usual either. Which job in the 21st century doesn't have long working hours, high levels of stress, or a lack of work-life balance? I can't think of a single one. So basically, I was barred from going back to my previous fast-paced, high-pressure work life with long hours and no boundaries or balance. I needed to figure out how I'd find new opportunities having already announced to the world my medical condition, knowing very well there would limited opportunities that would be available to me because people have their own biases about what a brain cancer survivor can and cannot do.

In the past, I had always envied those who worked as freelancers, gig workers, or part-time consultants. I imagined they got the best of both worlds—money for their fixed/limited hours of work and time to do as they pleased. Sure, the pay was lesser, there was no guaranteed monthly income, and no official titles that could show any growth. But equally, there would be neither unrealistic expectations, unnecessary stress, nor soul-crushing work hours. Plus, this form of working would allow me to take care of my health, get the doctor-prescribed afternoon naps, and work on my passion projects in the evening. All in all, it sounded perfect. I could do a part-time or freelance day job that covered my expenses and do a meaningful evening project that was fulfilling. That is precisely how I worked on this book while working as a remote part-time learning and development head at a diversity and inclusion firm during the day, conducting freelance virtual training sessions when possible in the late afternoons, and organizing and writing this book in the evenings and over weekends. I feel like I have found the perfect fit for myself, for now. But deciding what to do both in the morning and evening was still a struggle.

I studied media and communication as an undergraduate student, worked in advertising briefly only to be completely disillusioned, and transitioned to education, skill development, and training. I then spent almost seven years in this space—building skills, credibility, and a portfolio. I even got into a master's program in the same field at Harvard University. But now I was questioning if I wanted to continue doing this in whatever time I had left. Clearly, I was having another career crisis, just like the one I had had at the beginning of my career.

I entered this field because I'm really passionate about helping others. What better way to do it than through education and training. My own education at two of the finest educational institutions in the country (St. Xavier's College, Mumbai, and Ashoka University, Delhi NCR) had given me fantastic exposure, personal growth, and cognitive-social-emotional skills. They made me the person I am today. While not everyone can study at these places due to the inequities that exist in the system, I strongly believe that building

21st-century skills through technology can make a huge difference. That's the potential I saw in Edtech that was catapulted to the forefront during the pandemic. However, as the pandemic subsided and folks started going back to schools, colleges, and workplaces, everyone seemed to be tired of virtual/online learning. Although touted to be the next game changer in education, I wasn't sure if there was any future in the field. But I know there would always be cases where remote/blended/hybrid learning would be the only option that works for working professionals. Hence, I have decided to not completely abandon this field, especially working with adult learners. Building learning experiences and delivering them, both in-person and virtually, is something I'm really good at and love doing, so I shall continue working on them, albeit part-time and as a freelancer for now. This shall be one of my gigs in the portfolio career I intend to build for myself. That means, if my health permits, I'll go back to Harvard in the fall of 2023.

I'm also passionate about helping students navigate career options and apply to universities abroad. I've helped over a dozen of my friends make solid career decisions and apply and get through several universities abroad, including world's top 10-15 universities, with most of them in the Ivy League. So, I know how to work with people and understand them and their aspirations to be able to help them find their own paths. Maybe that'll be another gig that I will work on in the future. However, I also want to work on passion projects that'll help people in other areas of life. I'm a strong mental health advocate, and have trained as a coach. I've also started training to become a counselor. Maybe someday, I will finish those programs and give back to society. Getting this book written and published was another passion project. I hope to continue doing more of these, getting bigger and bolder with every project. The next one that I have my eyes set on is building the much-needed support system and resources for the Indian young adult cancer community.

I am also hoping that this portfolio career of part-time/freelance/gig opportunities will leave me with enough time and resources to engage in my hobbies and interests which I want to actively explore before it's too late—travel the world, try different cuisines, learn new dance forms, write more poetry, perform in front of large audiences, publish a memoir, and so on. My impairments and restrictions make it difficult to pursue several of these currently, but I am hoping with time and perhaps support, I'll be able to check these off my bucket list. All of these are currently works-in-progress, and I'm moving one step closer with each passing day. I'm confident that I'll eventually check off all the boxes.

One of the biggest traps, I have realized in less than a year of being diagnosed, is the urge to go back to "normal." I'm referring to the desire to go back to life and work as they were before all of this "happened" to you. Unfortunately, that's never going to happen. That life just doesn't exist anymore. Any attempt to replicate it, either by throwing yourself into work with the same gusto or living life at the same pace as before will only lead to exhaustion and trips to the hospital, reminding you that your body isn't the same anymore, so nor can your life or career be. I speak from personal experience—I tried to fill my days as I used to before treatment and I quickly realized that I was more tired and fatigued than I was even immediately after my surgery. My concentration and focus were completely off, and I had more seizures when I was stretching/ stressing myself. FOMO, the fear of missing out, is another trap that you will keep falling into a lot, looking at all that your friends and peers are doing and achieving in their personal and professional lives on social media—partying, traveling the world, climbing the career ladder, or being extremely successful according to what is considered the norm in society. Comparing myself to them only made me feel spiteful and less happy. So, I have been trying to avoid doing that, not always successfully. You are allowed to grieve the loss of all that you could be doing and would have been right now had cancer not happened to you. I've been mourning for almost a year now while continuing to live my life and trying to move forward. I don't know how long it will take for me to be completely over "it" or if I ever will. Know that you are not the only one who struggles with this.

Arriving at these conclusions wasn't easy at all. There was a lot of reflection, vision boarding, mind mapping, asking myself and people who know me what they thought I did well and could do for a living now and introspecting on what I would do if money wasn't a problem, which it obviously is, given how expensive cancer treatments are. However, for the sake of this exercise, let's imagine it isn't important. I also knew I would probably die sooner than later and what all I wanted to do before I did. These helped me come up with some options for both my day job as well as passion projects. In the spirit of transparency, all of this is still on a trial-and-error basis as it has been just a year since my treatment. Most of it has worked for me so far. However, I'm going to play it by the ear and pivot/adjust as and when needed, till I find something that works for me and keeps me happy. If I have limited time left, I certainly don't want to spend it all working. I don't want to regret not living when I had the chance. Who knows what deficits the next round of recurrence and subsequent treatments will bring? So, I focus on "seizing the day," while I continue engaging in meaningful work and play.

I know many cancer survivors who went back to what they were doing before right after their treatment and recovery. But that wasn't working for me earlier and wasn't an option anymore either, so I had no choice but to look for alternatives. I might still go back to full-time work after coming back from Harvard, albeit one that isn't too stressful and, offers flexibility and a good work-life balance. There is no single way to reimagine your life and recalibrate your career with/post cancer. What I did may or may not help you. If it does, that's fantastic. If it doesn't, keep trying. I hope you'll eventually find something that works for you. And if it doesn't, that's also fine. As Shah Rukh Khan says in Om Shanti Om, "Picture abhi baaki hai mere dost" (the movie is yet to end my friend).

—Sanjay Deshpande

EXPLORING
EXISTENTIAL
QUESTIONS

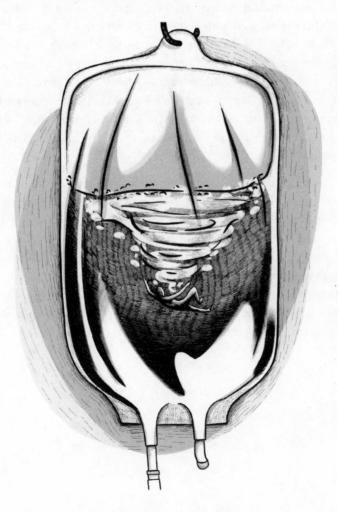

The minute we hear the word "cancer," we imagine the end of our lives because we have seen it happen in so many movies. Cancer is equated with certain death and this has created a taboo around it. No matter how treatable/curable it might be, we are bound to think about our mortality—the fact that we will eventually perish, perhaps earlier than expected. With this awareness, comes a certain sense of clarity about all that really matters to us, and we try to live a more authentic life, doing things that we find meaningful, which were earlier pushed to an uncertain future.

Cancer also ends up testing our faith. While some of us may stop believing, others start believing or remain unfettered. Some of us question the existence of a "benevolent god" for meting out this punishment to us, despite being a "devout" believer and living life as a "good person." For those of us who get cured, it cements our belief in the existence of a "divine" being who has a plan for us and has guided us through the whole ordeal. Read two starkly different perspectives on how cancer changes our worldview.

DANCING WITH DEATH

What is the first thing that would cross your mind if you heard, "You have cancer." All I could think of was death. I thought I was going to die soon. My entire life flashed in front of my eyes, and I became acutely aware of how fragile life truly is. Suddenly, I became conscious of my mortality to which I was otherwise oblivious. It's not that I thought I was immortal or invincible. I just didn't think much about dying and believed I had a long time before I would have to worry about it.

Since my diagnosis, I have spent a lot of time thinking about death and dying. It's a rite of passage for those who join the cancer club, one that nobody ever wants to be a part of. This preoccupation with death is common in the cancer world. It's impossible not to think about it. Some days you do it out of helplessness, seeking a modicum of control over your life. On others, you do it to try to make meaning of your suffering.

One of the paradoxes of being a cancer survivor is the fact that the whole experience makes you realize how easily and quickly your life can be snuffed out without any fault of your own. Yet, you can't often do much about it. We like to believe that we are the captains of our own ships, writers of our own destinies, and fate is for those who leave things to chance. While this may be valid to some extent, the ultimate truth is that we can't really control everything, no matter how much we would like to. Unpredictable things happen all the time. When it happens in nature like an earthquake, cyclone, or tsunami that kills people, we call them "an act of god." When something highly unusual and unlikely happens to an individual, something that kills them, we call it a "freak accident." But what about life-threatening diseases like cancer? They happen to a large number of people and are highly unusual and unlikely. So, do they qualify as an "act of god" or "freak accidents"?

One might argue that some of them are preventable—avoiding or quitting smoking can significantly reduce the chances of getting mouth and lung cancer. Sometimes it is due to environmental factors like air pollution; you could choose to live somewhere with clean air. It might even be due to hereditary factors—you might have a high genetic risk of developing it, so you follow all the precautions to avoid it. Now, despite controlling all that you possibly could, if you still get cancer, who can you blame? I grappled with these questions in the first few months after my treatment.

After my surgery, I was working with a yoga teacher to recover physically since I needed to exercise but wasn't allowed to do anything vigorous. The doctors had warned me against being sedentary or bed-bound. My teacher also taught Vedantic scriptures. So, for a brief period of time, I tried to find answers to my existential questions in spirituality. I read Eastern and Western philosophies extensively in the hopes of finding some answers. Luckily, I found a few.

Humans like control and certainty, two things nature does not always afford us. The whole premise of all spiritual practices is this: we tend to falsely believe that we are in control and can control what happens to us. We fear death when death is the ultimate truth, an inevitable end to our journey. So, the sooner we make peace with death, the sooner we truly start living. Some suggest there is an afterlife, some say you may be reborn. The undeniable truth is that no matter which school of practice you follow, there is no escaping death.

At one point, I took to existentialism to find solace. I'm agnostic, so I found it easier to accept that humans are just another step in the evolution of our planet. Many species came before us and many will perhaps come after unless we destroy our planet to such an extent that we make it unlivable. While we might want to accord meaning to our existence and live long, healthy, and fulfilling lives, life is inherently meaningless and at the mercy of luck. If you are born with the right genes in the right family and in the right location, you might grow up healthy, achieve success, and prosper—you might even live a long life given your access to superior healthcare. But if you didn't, you wouldn't even be able to access life-saving medicines and treatments. I think about this all the time. I was able to get excellent treatment because I have a lot of privilege—I'm a cisgendered, able-bodied, middle-class, upper caste, English educated, postgraduate from the top Indian colleges with a financial safety net. Not to forget the special access I get for having parents who are both doctors. I shudder at the thought of what I would have done otherwise.

In his seminal essay "Pale Blue Dot," Carl Sagan, the famous astrophysicist, discussed the Earth being just one tiny spec in the cosmos consisting of billions of planets, stars, and galaxies. So, all those we know, love, and care about today and all those who ever lived on this tiny dot, will eventually go or have gone back to being stardust, back to where we came from. There is something about the vastness of space and the largeness of the cosmos that humbles you and puts your life into perspective. Yes, you have cancer and might be staring at potential death. Yes, you are giving it your all and holding onto the hope that you might overcome this. But, would your death really make any difference to anyone? Sure, it will affect those who love and care about you, but the world doesn't stop and will keep moving. You'll perhaps not even be remembered once everyone who knows you dies as well. If that's the case, why do we fear death so much? Is it the lack of significance that scares us? Is that why we want to leave legacies behind so that we will be remembered? Or is it the uncertainty of what lies on the other side? What if there is no other side? Does the finality of death scare us? I believe it is all of that and more.

I'm currently not in active treatment. This means I'm currently tumor-free but there is a possibility of it growing back sometime in the future. Relapse, recurrence, and metastasis are real dangers for anyone who has had cancer, even if they have been completely cured. I am currently under observation, being monitored regularly for any change in my status. My life now revolves around tests and hospital visits. Time is measured as the intervals between my MRI scans. Each upcoming scan gives me sleepless nights. In the cancer community, this phenomenon is called scanxiety. God! It's so debilitating. Just as I recover from my last scan and get some semblance of normalcy back, the next one is right around the corner. I'm chained to my doctors for the rest of my life. Mind you, I'm not ungrateful for all that they do, but I feel like a bird trapped in a cage, free to live only within the confines of my mandatory MRI scans, hospital visits, and recommended restrictions.

There is a sword hanging over my head that constantly reminds me of my mortality. In some ways, it nudges me to live life more urgently, one day at a time. Savoring each moment. Storing good memories for the difficult times that may lie ahead. Doing things that have been on my bucket list but which were pushed for later, assuming that I would have a "later," and enough time and energy to do them. So, the only silver lining that I have been able to find through this entire experience is that cancer made me recalibrate my priorities and helped me do things I have always wanted to do, and do them now. I wanted to write poetry, so I started writing it. I even performed spoken word poetry at an event, receiving a standing ovation. I wanted to be a published author, so I decided to lead the effort to write and get this book published. I couldn't possibly write an entire book alone, not yet at least. So, envisioning this book and writing a few chapters was my way of preparing to write the memoir that is on my bucket list. I also wanted to become a coach/therapist, so I joined and completed level one of a training program to be one. No more procrastinating and keeping things for later. I am literally carpe diem-ing my way through life. Seizing each day as perhaps my last has made a huge difference to how I live. This is not to say that every day is a good day. I struggle with depressive episodes as much as any other cancer patient, but I try to not let them take over whatever time I have left.

I have lost a lot of family members over the course of my life. My maternal grandaunt passed away right after my brain surgery. Her death affected me deeply. She had inspired me to dream big and pursue my passion for education but she had been suffering for a long time. When she died of a heart attack during a routine checkup, my father asked me to rush to the hospital she was in. I walked into the ER where her pale body was lying motionless. My mother was weeping next to her. I tried to console her while I cried silently. But I noticed something peculiar—she finally seemed at peace, not suffering anymore. I will never be able to forget that sight. It's permanently etched into my memory. Her son lived in the US so we had to keep her in a morgue till he was able to fly down to India. On the day we performed her last rites, I brought her back. Seeing her being extracted from the freezer at the morgue, being transferred into the ambulance, and then sitting next to the driver while her cold, slowly decaying body lay right behind me as we drove through the city, I couldn't help but wonder who would be the person carrying my body and conducting my last rites if I were in her place. Would it be my father? I imagine myself in his shoes and feel indescribable pain and grief. In the natural order, it's supposed to be the other way round—I being the one doing his rites, not him. What if I passed away after him or both my parents—would it then be my only paternal male cousin or my brother-in-law who does my last rites? If it ever comes to that, I hope it's my sister who lights my funeral pyre, to hell with Indian customs and traditions.

Later, after mourning my grandaunt's death, when I was finally able to process what had happened, I realized that looking at her finally at peace erased my fear of death. I was no longer scared of dying anymore. However, in the spirit of honesty, this doesn't mean I'm not scared anymore. I'm still scared of a painful or prolonged death and of dying alone. If there is any supernatural entity out there, my only prayer to them is to give me as much time as I can get with a good quality of life with my loved ones and a quick and painless death. I don't care much about living long if that means suffering as a result of it. But I do care about how I'm able to live while I'm still alive and how I'd like to be treated if I'm on my deathbed.

I have spent many sleepless nights wondering who will take care of my aging parents just in case I pass away before them. I know my sister will be there for them in the best possible way she can, but she lives in the US. Coming from a traditional middle-class family, my parents invested heavily in my education, hoping it will help me make a career and live independently. While they have never expected any financial help, I knew that I would eventually have to support them once the two of them are unable to work. Since both of them have finally "retired," I now acutely sense the need to earn and provide for them, for as long as I can. As they have grown older, I have also had to play referee when they have had arguments or fights, and even had to counsel and teach them how to deal with people, build friendships, mend relationships, order food online, book cabs, manage finances, and take better care of their own health. Oh, how the tables have turned! In some ways, I have become the parent and they have become the child. I often wonder what they would do if I wasn't around anymore.

In our culture, we don't discuss end-of-life decisions at all. We would rather let the person suffer in their final days than talk about what to do if they were dying and unable to communicate or make sound decisions anymore. No matter how uncomfortable it made my parents, I have been quite vocal about what my wishes are, even before I was wheeled in for my surgery. Brain surgery is quite dangerous in itself but can be more threatening when trying to remove a tumor. I remember telling my father quite sternly that if the doctor came out mid-surgery to ask if they would like him to continue removing my tumor if there was a risk of leaving lasting deficits, he would tell the neurosurgeon only to remove as much as was safe to remove without causing deficits. I was willing to take my chances with other treatments like chemotherapy and radiation if some of the tumor was left behind, but not with a compromised quality of life.

I still maintain the same position. I would rather live a full life and die early than live longer but suffer more. I have also told them that if there ever came a time to keep me on the ventilator, I don't want to be on it unless there was a 100% guarantee that it would help me, and certainly not for more than a week. I do not want to be kept alive using machines. The same is true in case I have a heart attack. I do not want to be resuscitated. I would rather have a sudden death than a painful, protracted one. Some might say that's extreme. Well, it's how I would like to live and die, and I believe everyone has to be given the right to choose these things. I am not denying that this might be an impossible situation for my family, but I really hope that they will respect my wishes, if and when the time comes. I want to be remembered as the happy and high-spirited person I am rather than the sickly and incapacitated one I will become if I am on a ventilator or resuscitated from a heart attack.

Death is the final frontier, one that none of us can escape from. Mortality is our true reality, yet we often ignore, deflect, reject, forget, and hide from it. Let's just say, as a brain cancer survivor, I had no way out but to reflect on it and accept it.

—Sanjay Deshpande

RELIGION, FAITH
AND CANCER

Asatoma Sad Gamaya
Tamasoma Jyotir Gamaya
Mrityurma Amritam Gamaya
Om Shanti Shanti Shanti Hi

[O Mother lead me from falsehood to Truth
From Darkness to Light
From Death to Immortality
Let there be Peace, Peace, Peace]

—Pavamana Mantra, Brihadaranyaka Upanishad (1.3.28)

Religion is the opium of the masses, but...
—Karl Marx

As a cancer patient raised in an atmosphere dominated by Left-leaning academia, these two verses might aptly describe my tryst with religion. While Marx's often repeated and abused quote is ingrained into the minds of innocent newcomers entering the hallowed halls of academia by teachers, seniors, friends, and "Red flag"—obsessed student organizations, any life-threatening disease or near-death experience often forces some Leftists to revisit their notions of religion or faith. This reckoning and feeling of nihilistic confusion may lead one to find solace in the Pavamana Mantra quoted above. It was similar to how I felt during my struggle with Chronic Myeloid Leukemia (CML). After being diagnosed, I had a rush of emotions and feelings such as confusion and fear. I landed on the Pavamana Mantra because I was in dire need of someone (whether human or supernatural power) who would lead me from darkness to light and from ignorance to knowledge about my condition. The most important one for me was the part "*mrityurma amritam gamaya*" or the desire to transcend mortality and death at a time when Yama, the god of death, was staring at me. Yet, as they say in the Tibetan book *Badro Thodol* (Book of the Dead) about death not being the end, or the dialogue by Sun God Ra (portrayed by Geoffrey Rush) in the 2016 movie *Gods of Egypt* which says, "Immortality awaits us only in the afterlife. Our entire journey in this life is to prepare us for the afterlife." I too thought about my immortality post my demise. My fears were allayed solely after listening to the words of my Guruji (my professor at Ashoka University) who asked me to keep calm and have faith in the Devi (Mother Goddess) who is the beginning and the end of all and who is beyond as well as within every being and object in the cosmos. As per him, the Devi must have had something in mind to have "blessed" or inflicted me with the disease which would be revealed later. When he mentioned that his niece too had been through a similar travail but of a much more serious nature, that too in the 1990s when medical science had not advanced to the current level, and yet had emerged successful, I got a semblance of belief in myself and the faith in the Devi. I too hoped to succeed.

When I was admitted to a hospital for the first time in my life and that too for a period of two weeks, my level of hope and strength plummeted as I lay in the bed staring at the walls with only the occasional visits from the nurse to check my BP, take blood samples, measure weight, and remove the connection between the peripherally inserted central catheter (PICC) line attached to my hand and the bag administering chemotherapy whenever I had to answer the call of nature. It was also because for the first time in my life, I was confined to a bed and a few walls with nowhere to walk or gallivant around. Although I had occasional visits and received phone calls from relatives and friends, who would often strongly encourage me to not lose faith and maintain my inner strength, they often appeared patronizing or preachy. Sometimes these words of encouragement felt learned by rote. Like a parrot they were repeating the same thing over and over again, as I was sinking deeper and deeper into the quagmire of hopelessness, weakness, and pessimism.

However, an event shook me up from my spiritual laziness and slumber. My mother, who had arrived to take her position as my attendant after my father had left, told me in an excited voice about her visit to the Shirdi Sai Temple in Delhi before coming to the hospital. As per the daily rituals, the idol of Sai Baba was bathed and cleaned and new clothes were put on it. It so happened that on the day my mother paid a visit, the cloth which she had bought as an offering to Sai Baba was the first cloth and offering to be given, and hence the idol was dressed in those clothes. On seeing this, the priest remarked to my mother that it was a sign of Sai Baba having accepted her prayers and that her son would soon recover. As she placed the yellow-colored cloth given by the temple priest beneath my pillow and sprinkled the *vibhuti* (ash) of Shirdi Sai on my face, I felt a sparkle of hope and life arise within me. These "sacred objects" together with the event narrated by my mother made me question whether it was just a coincidence according to the Left rationalist inside me or was it something more—a message emanating from the cosmos or the Divine itself?

As Master Oogway said to his disciple Shifu in *Kung Fu Panda*, "Who knows the ways of the universe? Accident or destiny? That is the secret." Maybe, the believer in me liked to believe it was a sign that the Divine was with me—a supernatural being such as the Devi, God, Allah, or Yahweh (depending on your religious affiliation) who went beyond the speculations of the human mind and appeared at times only to underline the fragility of human rationality and logic, especially to individuals like me steeped in the Marxian "iron cage" (borrowing from Max Weber, a German sociologist) or Red bars.

Sometimes, I wonder whether the Marxian bars or the "Red" colored cages were not actually manufactured or built by Marx

himself but his followers who either deliberately or out of ignorance only focused on the first half of his statement, "Religion is
the opium of the masses, but..." It is the following "but" that is
often brushed under the carpet in Marxist study circles or in Left
stronghold institutions. It goes like this—"but the heart of the heart-
less world." Although I will be attacked by the class warriors armed
with their Red holy books for daring to "desecrate" one of their
most sacred commandments, yet I would like to say that no matter
what turns the tide of history takes (based on one's belief), there
was, is, and has always existed, a power beyond us and within all of
us which permeates the entire cosmos. A belief in the said power
should not be imposed, or forcefully shoved down people's throats
through the fear of hell, eternal punishment, *paap* (sin), or the use
of violence. It has to be felt, experienced, and then accepted by individuals themselves. The Bhakti and Sufi saints of our subcontinent
such as Mahapurush Srimanta Sankardeva, Meera Bai, Hathiram
Vairagi, Ajan Fakir, Nizamuddin Auliya, and Rashkan are a case
in point. They became *mahatmas/auliyas* (great souls) and *bhaktas/
bhaktins* (devotees) not because they blindly followed or uncritically
accepted what the society taught them. Instead, they felt and experienced *prem/ishq* (love) for the Divine on their own accord. The
entire episode with cancer was in a way a moment of the revelation
of the Divine for me. I felt as if a divine strength nudged me on
and didn't allow me to give up. It was through these circumstances
that I discovered the Divine. This new devotion for the Divine was
not imposed on me by some quack claiming the cancer to be a
sign of God's displeasure with my irreverence. Rather, the Divine,
I believe, had struck me with the disease in order to make me realize and cherish the value of things that I had since then taken for
granted—family, friends, society, and most importantly faith.

Along with the prayers performed by my mother and our family priest in Haridwar, my father's friend had donated a *chaadar*
(cloth) in my name in Mecca, and another friend of my father had
asked him to apply *amrit* or water from the Gurudwara on me every
day and my sister-in-law had blessed me with a Bible reading in

Guwahati before my departure for Delhi. It seemed as if the Gods of all major religions were being invoked to cure me. Hence, while I believed myself to be the subject of divine favor, at the same time I thought I too shouldered a responsibility not to go down into hopelessness or lose faith for the prayers to work. After all, it's a two-way traffic as "God helps those only who help themselves." My journey with cancer thus far has been a mutually reinforcing relationship between faith (in God and oneself) and divine aid which I call "spiritual medicine." To me, it is as important as "secular medicine" or scientific medical treatment. Secular and spiritual medicine are not mutually exclusive. Instead, they reinforce each other. Secular or scientific medication would not work if one gives up the will to live and fight and withdraws into a pessimistic mode. Or, in other words, they wouldn't work if one does not try to harness one's mind to heal as a result of having given up hope. For instance, as per traditional Tibetan medicine, the mind (or inner strength) also plays an important role in healing or degradation along with medical treatment. On the other hand, a complete and blind reliance on spiritual medicine or prayers and healings without the assistance of secular medicine is not only foolhardy but also fatal. According to the Tibetan tradition, during specific and serious illnesses such as cancer one must chant and meditate upon the Buddhist deity *Black Manjushri* asking for his divine intervention to fight the demon (cancer) but at the same time, the meditation must be accompanied by medical treatment at the hospital. Now the question arises: how does one go about strengthening spiritual medicine? Along with belief and faith, I also did *dhyana* (meditation) and yoga, especially *pranayama* (yogic breathing exercises), which allowed me to keep my mind calm and maintain my confidence.

In the weekly appointments post my initial release in April 2021, the daily reports gave an indication of the lessening number of platelet count and hemoglobin. When the numbers went too low, bordering on serious complications, I was sometimes admitted for two days or a week. Those were the times when I would question my faith and my confidence would waver as I saw my father running from pillar to post to obtain donors for the hospital blood bank. My confidence further dropped when I was diagnosed with COVID-19 and I earned a new epithet, "comorbid." My mind buzzed with numerous questions and doubts. I had this burning urge to know, out of all the people whom I had encountered back in my home-town as well in the hospital, was I the one to be cursed with this disease? Why didn't God or the pandemic strike those who had openly flouted the COVID-19 norms and shown the middle finger to doctors and government protocols with the declaration "my body my rules"? All these lingering doubts worsened my condition, although my father kept nudging me not to lose hope. Despite his best efforts, my condition didn't improve and I was admitted to the hospital in the second week.

Once I was admitted to the COVID-19 ward, my fear of death increased as I saw myself surrounded by patients mostly in their 70s and 80s attached to various kinds of breathing machines, oxygen cylinders, and life support systems. I shuddered at the thought that I would be in a similar situation as them. Seeing my face becoming pale with fright, my father refused to leave me until the doctor came. Looking into my eyes, the doctor simply said, "If you keep looking at the other patients, it will only add to your fears and worsen your illness. Hence, keep in mind that they belong to a different age group and you have the advantage of being younger and possessing a comparatively higher oxygen capacity than them." Though these words did not completely allay my fears, they gave me some respite and an inkling of hope that I might make it. But the power of those words was such that although I had witnessed a patient passing away and his body being wrapped for cremation, I felt no fear and instead prayed for a peaceful afterlife for him and for his family to find the strength to bear the grim news. On the fourth day, I was transferred to a personal ward, away from my fellow geriatric patients. It was here that my mind gradually stopped dwelling on death. I noticed that as I slowly drew my attention away from the virus, I was getting more hopeful and my body was showing signs of recovery. All this while I kept doing my *dhyan* and *pranayama* and finally at the end of the second week I was allowed to go home. During this ordeal, were the doctor's words in the COVID-19 ward a sign from the Divine not to give up? Did my belief in the Divine despite my mind teeming with doubts and questions lead to my recovery? Or was I inflicted with COVID-19 so that I could learn the lesson of not giving up as well as the importance of spiritual medicine (*dhyan*, *pranayama*, and belief in oneself)? I don't have the answers.

My next experience of the marriage between spiritual and secular medicine came during the Bone Marrow Transplant (BMT) in September 2021 and the harrowing days that followed. At the onset, the doctor along with the nurses said a short prayer and post the transplant, the doctor said that the completion of the procedure was akin to a *punarjanam* (rebirth) for me. Although I was quite scared about the BMT, it turned out to be the most painless process I was subjected to during the course of my treatment. The real reckoning came in the weeks following the BMT. First, it began with the depletion of hemoglobin and platelet count and gradually a drop in appetite. Despite that, I kept force-feeding myself to the extent I could and kept drinking water. I found myself in the same situation as when I was first admitted in March with the same level of low energy and enthusiasm. Add to that the fact that I wasn't even allowed to step out of my room in the BMT ward to avoid infection. Although during the BMT process the doctor had warned me about the consequences, such as a drop in blood cell counts, fever, diarrhea, and even boils or ulcers on the tongue in the initial few weeks or months, I thought that I would easily sail through given the support I had from the Divine. The moment of doubt returned when the problem of piles and hemorrhoids resurfaced (I was inflicted with them post COVID-19). They left me with intense and sometimes unbearable pain during and post bowel movements. Sometimes, they gave me sleepless nights and I would often be forced to think would it have been better had I not undergone BMT. Whenever the doctor visited, I always asked the same question as to when could I scoot free from this "prison," only to be told that some of my co-patients (as young as six-year-olds) had been staying in the ward for three to four months while I was already complaining in my second week. The persistent piles, loss of appetite, and the confinement to a room with only a window that connected me to the outside world only worsened my fears of being trapped there for four or more months. However, the Divine also expressed its support for me through the encouraging words of the nurse who said that as compared to other patients a positive sign from my side was that at least I was gobbling food and water even after two weeks. The other patients were trapped in the ward because of their inability to consume anything given the presence of ulcers on their tongue and throat. They were being fed through saline lines. Thank God I did not develop ulcers at least. Was it another indication from the Divine that I should stop complaining and be thankful that I was in a better position as compared to the other patients?

The "compliment" from the nurse ignited some hope that I would get out of the hospital soon. Meanwhile, my mother advised me to listen to *Vishnu Sahasranamam* (the 1000 names of Lord Vishnu) while falling asleep as it would soothe my pain. It did work sometimes, although not always. Yet after a few days, I was slowly regaining my old self as I would eat comparatively more than earlier and also began to harness the power of my spiritual medicine through *dhyana and pranayama* as well as listening to *strotams* and *stutis* (chants and verses in praise of God). The effects of my spiritual medicine, which I believe also began affecting my internal body processes, was seen in the slowly climbing blood counts and other gradual slow-paced improvements. Finally, after having spent 24 days in the BMT ward, I was released in a wheelchair to the cheers and claps of the nurses as well as staff members.

What did I learn from these experiences? I believe they taught me not to lose hope and go on without giving up. As they say, perseverance is the key. I think the Divine put me through these tests in order to steel my resolve. Whether through the Sai temple incident, the words of the COVID-19 ward doctor, or the encouragement of the nurse in the BMT ward, the Divine often sent signs to let me know that I was not alone.

As I write this chapter, I am not sure whether I have truly become a *bhakt* (in the religious sense) or a true believer. As Swami Leeladhar (portrayed by Mithun Chakraborty) says to Kanji (portrayed by Paresh Rawal) in the 2012 movie *Oh My God* (OMG), "They are not God-loving people, they are God-fearing people," implying how it was easy to fool and exploit the masses in the name of religion and through the fear of God and hell as shown in the movie (and hence the Leftist dictum of opium of the masses). Has the experience with leukemia made me love God because of the Divine support which I believe I had throughout the challenging days? Or have I become God-fearing, living in an unknown fear of incurring divine wrath by committing the silliest of mistakes such as entering the temple without having taken a bath? I am not sure. Perhaps I have not been able to get rid of my fear of death or mortality as since the BMT. I often shudder whenever I hear the news of anyone's passing away or someone being in an accident or getting diagnosed with a certain illness. The fear which grabs me is whether I would have to face such a fate for any minor transgression on my part. But at the same time, my experience has also made me empathetic and more understanding of those who are facing a similar ordeal. Hence, even if I am not able to contribute medically or financially, I always pray in the hope that similar to the way it gave me signs and showed me the path to spiritual strength, the Divine would do the same for those who are facing a similar crisis. After all, isn't service to others service to God?

Finally, which explanation do I accept? Were the above anecdotes something emanating from the cosmos or just a chain of lucky coincidences? Was I favored by Divine grace or did I just encounter an illusion in the face of the unacceptability of the fragility of life? Am I trying to be a new thug Baba like Mithun *da's* Leeladhar by converting Red comrades to my belief system through this chapter? Or am I just stating what I felt throughout this ordeal? For believers, am I a God-loving or God-fearing person? You decide. I am no *acharya*, *saint*, or *wali* (holy men) here to convert you. You may or may not decide to feel the Divine yourself. I am not going to command you or else I am no better than bigots making cameos in newspapers and televisions. As Gautam Buddha said, *Apo Deepo Bhava* (be your own light).

—Anuraag Khaund

FINANCE, INSURANCE, AND HOSPITALS

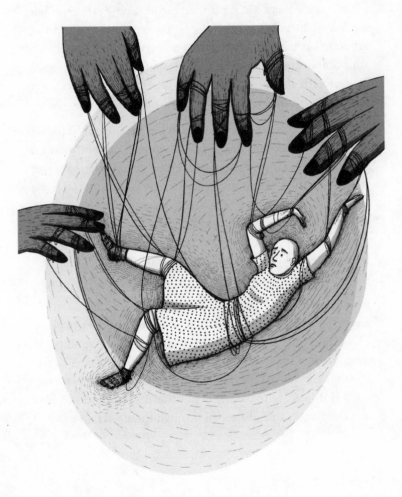

Cancer is an expensive and dangerous disease. Siddhartha Mukherjee, an Indian-American physician, biologist, and author, calls it "the emperor of all maladies" for good reason. It can squeeze every ounce of health, happiness, and hard-earned money from a patient/survivor and their caregivers, often leaving them worse off than earlier. Some get better but are left financially insecure. Some neither get better and nor are they left with any funds. Several people have gone bankrupt due to the expensive medicines and treatments needed to deal with this insidious illness. One often wonders what happens to those who can't afford treatment.

Insurance plays a life-saving role. It helps tide over the ordeal in an already stressful time without worrying about finances. However, insurance claims are another battle. Not to forget that if one didn't have insurance before the treatment, there isn't a single practical one available that will actually help in times of need. So, one is left financially vulnerable for the rest of one's life, often even unable to bear other non-cancer-related medical expenses that one may incur.

The other bane is having to navigate the bureaucratic hospital system. While it is mostly logistics, it can be really annoying and punch a huge hole in an individual's pockets. The innumerable follow-up tests, scans, and visits, and being made to wait for hours to meet one's doctor for barely a few minutes can make one lose faith in the whole process, especially if things aren't getting better. Read on to find out how some of our co-authors waded through these wild forests.

I belong to the school of writing where every story must have an exotic setting. Mine is set in Finland in the year 2014 when I was an exchange student. My experience was postcard perfect except for a small wound, which, thanks to my foolhardiness, turned into a full-blown pus-filled abscess. Whoever received lemons from life has been really lucky, because it's mostly been brinjals in my basket. Predictably, my abscess decided to burst two days before I was scheduled to leave Finland. As I sat on a bus, leaking blood and pus, it still hadn't sunk in that I may have to seek medical attention. My Finnish friend, who was training to be a midwife at the time, dressed my wound as best as she could, and we decided to wait and watch. The next morning, my wound was still leaking so we decided to go to a clinic. The doctor took a look and referred me to a big hospital. The fact that my wound emitted an odor might give you an idea about how badly my wound was infected. I don't think everyday wounds are supposed to smell. So off to the hospital we went.

At the big hospital, I waited for the on-duty doctor to become available while the anesthesia kicked in. For a brief moment, the abscess became bearable. Next thing I knew, the doctor was prodding around my wound while I tried not to show any signs of weakness. In my mind, I was representing my country, and we are not a nation of weaklings. After all, I was a grown-up now. Once my wound was dressed, I was told I could leave. No hefty bill, thanks to socialism! *Kiitos paljon!* Thanks a lot!

Fast forward to a few months later—a hefty bill in Euros shows up at my house in Bengaluru. By this point, I had already returned to university to continue my studies. My dad called me, asking what the hell was happening. That's when I remembered I had bought insurance during the exchange trip. I had no idea whether they would accept it, but I filed a claim anyway. I can't stress enough how cumbersome it was. Zeus should have just made Sisyphus file an insurance claim for eternity. It's almost as if the process is the punishment for making them pay for your treatment. But as they say, all's well that ends well. The insurance company paid for my

RICH MAN'S DISEASE

If you have tried to watch something on YouTube recently,
might be familiar with this—you click play and suddenly there
video or a picture of a baby and there's someone crying and ask
for help. If this sounds familiar, what you have encountered
campaign video trying to raise funds for medical treatment. At t
point, you may click "skip ad" or choose to donate. No judgemer
here. I belonged to the "skip ad" gang until the day I found mys
having to think about starting a campaign to raise funds for n
own treatment. If you have read the book this far, you know that
presents the experiences of cancer survivors and patients, so I won
spend too much time on setting the context of my illness, excep
to say that I had it and now had to potentially raise money to trea
it. And raise lots of it. Like enough to buy a small apartment in
Bengaluru and a fairly big one in Timbuktu.

If my real estate comparisons are not painting a clear picture, let
me get into the numbers. At one point during my treatment, we
were looking at having to raise up to thirty-five lakhs for a specialized treatment. I hope you're drinking a beverage at this point so
you can spit it out for dramatic effect. Yes, specialized treatments
for cancer are *that* expensive. In fact, I have also seen a treatment
fundraiser with the target of over one crore. Turns out, fighting for
your life is expensive. I know what you're thinking. That's why you
should buy insurance, silly. I have insurance and it didn't help me.
In the interests of being fair, I will start my story by talking about
the time that insurance did help me.

very expensive Finnish misadventure. This experience taught me the importance of buying insurance, which is a lesson I have carried to this day.

The common perception is that young people don't buy insurance because they think they are infallible, but I haven't had the luxury of feeling that way because I have been in and out of hospitals since I was 14. I have always been aware that one needs money for medical expenses. So, the first thing I did when I started earning a decent salary was buy medical insurance. The amount of cover I bought at that time seemed like overkill, but I have now learned the very difficult lesson that medical treatments for conditions like cancer are obscenely expensive. I want to preface the rest of the chapter by saying that I have been extremely fortunate, even privileged, because I have always been able to afford treatment. But this isn't about me. It is about a systemic problem. How big is the problem? Let's break it down.

The till starts to clink the moment you walk into the hospital. In my case, this was in 2021. I had just collapsed after cycling and had rushed to the hospital to find out why. To get an answer to this "why," I had to get into an MRI machine. Thus began the tab. An MRI costs anywhere between fourteen to sixteen thousand rupees at a private hospital. So far in my cancer journey, I have had about six MRIs. Nearly every hospital we visited for opinions has taken an MRI scan of me. Adding CT scans, biopsies, tests, and consultations, the tab for just diagnostics has more zeros than is acceptable in an industry trying to save lives. I know what you're thinking. The smart writer told us a while back that he had bought insurance, so the very nice insurance company must have paid for all this. If only this was that kind of story. Gather around, kids, Grampy has a fun fact for you. Insurance does not pay for diagnostic tests, unless the test is being performed as a part of the surgery package. It doesn't pay for OPD consultations either

So, who pays for it? The patient. Well, mostly his parents. I have been able to afford all this thanks to my dad, who has paid for most of these tests. But I have to admit, it doesn't feel great seeing my dad pay for my treatments. Being a loving parent, he doesn't even think about it for a second, but deep down, I can't help feeling this sense of guilt. In the words of my therapist, let's explore this guilt further. I have thought a lot about why I feel guilty about something that is saving my life. I think it is partly because I earn my own salary now. I don't make figures worth bragging on LinkedIn about, but I do decently considering my college's name only had five letters in it. Somewhere deep inside my mind (amygdala and insula), there pops up a little thought that I really should be able to pay for my own treatment. Of course, the cerebrum knows that this is not a realistic expectation because I'm barely 30 and have only been working for four years. Even if I saved every single paisa I have made in my career so far, I would still not be able to pay for cancer treatment. But tetanus shots, I've got them covered! When you let it run amok, guilt can take you to some pretty dark places. At my lowest, I used the word "burden" to describe myself. What helped me overcome guilt was talking. Whenever these feelings crept up, I spoke to my partner or my sister and they both helped me see what my cerebrum already knew—I was being too hard on myself. I'm not the one charging so much money for life saving treatments, it was the hospitals.

Speaking of hospitals, my cancer journey also took me to one of India's largest government hospitals that undoubtedly has some of the best doctors in the world but the scenes there were dreary. The masses huddle outside from six in the morning, waiting to pay the consultation charges through a grill. There is of course the option to book a slot and pay online, but do you think this is a viable option for everyone? Then comes the waiting. There are hundreds of people waiting to see a doctor. If the doctor recommends that you need an MRI, then there is more waiting. No one can tell you for sure how long it will take. You wait till your name is called and hopefully you have all the right documents, otherwise, it's back to another building. Once you get to the counter, they ask you whether the patient needs to be restrained or is in control. You think to yourself why on earth would they ask you this. Then, you step into an MRI machine and realize why. It feels like you're in a coffin just below the earth's surface while earth-moving equipment is being driven just above. If you're a big, fidgety person like me, it is all the nine circles of hell. At the hospital, you see someone walking around with no life in their eyes or someone who can't move from the neck down and you say a little prayer hoping that's not you in the future. It's not uncommon to hear the staff being rude to someone who has probably traveled for days to be there. You wish they were a little kinder, but if you saw so many people with so many ailments day in and day out, you might treat people this way too. What I'm telling you might not come as a surprise. We are a developing nation and like many of our problems, this one also boils down to one simple truism—there are far too many of us and very few resources. But still, no one experiencing a life threatening illness should have to go through this while seeking affordable healthcare.

I am privileged enough that I could choose to undergo treatment at a private hospital. When the time came for my surgery, I had to play a nerve-wracking game of claim roulette as I wasn't sure whether my claim would be accepted or not. My own insurance company had refused to pay for my treatment because, wait for it, there was a waiting period of two years. In theory, it makes sense that insurance companies want to cover all their bases while insuring someone, but in reality, cancer cannot wait. Even a potentially dangerous tumor requires immediate removal. Suppose you bought insurance a year ago and need cancer treatment immediately, the insurer wishes you good luck and asks you to come back after two years. They even try to sell you a top-up while turning you down. When they said this to me, my reaction was similar to Brad Pitt's character Mickey in the movie *Snatch*. Simply put, "Why the f*** do I want a caravan that's got no fockin' wheels?!" Luckily for me, my employer also provided insurance. So, I placed my bet on the office insurance and I waited. Thankfully, the ball landed on the right number and they agreed to pay for my surgery, all eight lakhs of it.

From the time of my diagnosis, there was an expensive sword of Damocles hanging over my family's head due to the mention of a treatment called proton therapy. It sounds really fancy and it costs just as much. The moment I heard that I might have to undergo this treatment, I began thinking about how on earth we would raise thirty-five lakhs. I even started thinking about launching a fundraiser to raise money for my treatment. Fun fact: there are many platforms out there devoted solely to raising funds for medical treatment. Feels a lot like addressing the symptoms instead of the disease. At one point, I even told my sister that I would refuse treatment because I could not fathom raising and spending that much money on treatment. I felt that I would much rather take a loan and travel the world because that seemed like a better investment. My upper limit for self-worth is five lakhs max.

When is Marvel making Dad Man? In my story, Dad is the superhero. He and his friends from school would make pretty neat Avengers. They all offered to pitch in money for my treatment, no matter the cost. In the end, we found out that I didn't require the expensive treatment after all but could do with a much cheaper alternative. In the time between my surgery and my radiation treatment, I had just switched jobs, so it didn't feel right to claim medical insurance yet. So, my dad came to the rescue and mobilized funds for my treatment. At the time of writing this, I have completed my radiation treatment. All that remains now is regular follow-ups and MRIs for the next two years. Hopefully, the bastard doesn't come back.

As this chapter comes to a close, I would like to say that I have some solutions for all the things I told you are broken. But this isn't that kind of book and I'm not someone with answers, only thoughts. At best, I can tell you some things that I have learned during my treatment journey. Cancer is expensive to treat and those who aren't privileged or connected may not be able to get treatment. Insurance is useful but terms and conditions apply. Those are the bitter pills. Now for the lozenges. People can surprise you with their generosity and kindness. Life is hard, but people can and do make it easier. Many of the fundraisers you see on YouTube are actually successful and people do manage to get life saving treatments. It would be off-brand for me to end with a happy lesson, so I will end the chapter with this final one. Cancer patients find it difficult to buy insurance after being diagnosed, even if they have successfully undergone treatment. Even if you do get one, you have to pay more than the amount of coverage provided to buy it. Let that sink in.

–Aditya Arun

BATTLE TO FIGHT

I do not know much about cancer. It happened and left me no option but to undergo treatment.

In our shared vulnerabilities, my caregivers and I went with the flow. So, the simplistic identities projected onto me of being "brave" or a "warrior" seem ridiculous and disconnected from my reality. But if we are speaking of battles, I have a big one to fight—insurance.

I had insurance cover before cancer, but post cancer treatment I have none.

And guess what, I can't even get a new one. At present there are no useful insurance covers for people who have gone through or are living with cancer. I know well-meaning folks will point to certain starry insurance covers being offered, but I'll have to ask them to read the fine print. The gentleman selling it to me himself got embarrassed and apologized for suggesting it. Their extraordinarily high premiums and requirements that none of the ailments should be linked back to cancer or its treatment are atrocious and make them an absolute waste. One should rather invest in some funds. To illustrate my point, a dentist could link even a cavity to chemotherapy; swollen legs are linked to nerve damage during surgery (vague assumptions); liver disease is known to be caused by the specific chemo drugs used in my case. Similarly, there are so many other opportunistic infections and health conditions linked with cancer and its treatment. The bottom line is, I don't have a cover. I don't have much money either, and I spend a lot on my medical bills.

I worked hard since I was a child. I always performed well and scored high. I got through every institution I wanted to, and there, too, I worked hard and did well. Even though our family faced tragic experiences, I grew up with narratives of family and love that were particularly warm and helped me live with an illusion of safety. I am not sharing all of this to gain sympathy but to explain that in my perspective this wasn't the context for an insecure future. Is there ever a secure future? No, but one tries. I too had hopes of living a life with dignity. Dignity is precisely where I am stuck today.

I was diagnosed with cancer when I was slightly over thirty. I was planning to get married, rise in my career, and start building my savings. I am thirty-four and single now, my career is moving slowly as expected, and I am still spending on cancer. Long past my active treatment, I am now spending on follow-up scans, doctor visits, recurring infections, persistent side effects, medicines, hospital visits, iron infusions, and naive attempts at eating better food. Judging by the stereotypes around cancer observed on dating apps, I think my relationship status would remain the same for a while, not unlike my financial situation. I am mentioning both parallelly in the context of dignity because the fear of being alone makes everything much worse. It is not that I am truly alone; I have loving friends though they are mostly far away, my parents and my sibling do their best to be present, and I am grateful. Yet, deep inside a fear persists. I tried to avoid acknowledging that fear, resisting it with all my might, but when we hide from the truth, it comes out with greater force. This chapter is thus my attempt at being honest with myself and to you. I am not resisting anymore.

I once read that we are all one hospital visit away from poverty. The imagined future of financial destitution and physical limitations has shaken my boundaries of personal and collective responsibility. Be it health or even the requirements of daily life, I find myself awkwardly expecting help in goals that earlier were clearly mine to achieve. Even though I often stay hopeful, the fear of loneliness in this context slowly gnaws on my faith in life and in being self-reliant. Hence my ask for dignity. It has been close to four years since the ordeal began. A few weeks ago, I sent a rather paranoid text message to some of my friends, asking if they'll be there with me if I contracted other illnesses. Expecting another life to value mine so much, I am often taken aback by these expectations. I don't think it can be justified as my willingness to survive. It seems more like panic, driven by thoughts of living with illness. Dependence brings with it an anxiety of losing whatever support one has. It often reduces confidence. I have started seeking approvals and acknowledgements from those whose support I rely on. I find it hard to reclaim my own ideas of how I should be recovering and how I should be living my life because I am fearful. It is hard to live up to societal ideas of what is right for me. I had always courageously shunned those, but can I do so anymore, when this very society has helped in my treatment? Can I reclaim my right to privacy, financial independence, lifestyle, career, and health choices when my friends had raised funds for me? My resentment towards this loss of freedom actually offers me hope that a part of me is still alive. That I might just regain my muddled dignity.

Why do I mention these storms from my mind in a chapter on insurance? Because had I still had my insurance cover and had my prior expenses been covered by my insurance, I could have utilized my money to independently get the appropriate physical, emotional, and nutritional support I need right now rather than feel guilty or constantly worry about recurring and future medical expenses. I could have avoided the extreme distress in which my family members live ever since my treatment began because they do not find me calm, they see me wounded. Financial fears create confusion, but when combined with an enhanced understanding of our fragility and a reluctant admission of inevitable death, that too a lonely death, one without adequate support, the mix can be debilitating.

A friend had told me on the completion of my chemotherapy, "Now you shall begin, what could be perhaps, the loneliest part of this journey." Let alone the emotional upheavals, being on your own when you do not have appropriate money is absolute hardship. You call cancer treatment a battle? Welcome to cancer survival! It is perseverance; it requires will, yes. It requires a sense of meaning, yes. And it requires addressing panic, grief, and at times bitterness. I have been truly fortunate to be employed in this phase; I do not earn much because I do limited work. I have managed to spend on many of my needs but I cannot save right now. Not everyone can work in this phase. I am even more fortunate because I have caring colleagues and friends. Though fatigued, my parents and sibling accompany me on my journey. But my deep insecurity does not allow me to live in gratitude or stillness. I am more like a shaking Matryoshka doll (also known as a Russian Babushka doll, it is a wooden doll with tinier versions within). My outer self wants to be still, at peace with life, but there are anxious parts within wanting to come out.

I have identified three stages from my own journey:

Stage 1: No hope and reckless expenses. I only live in the present. Let me spend on making the present better. Let me make life easier for my loved ones by buying them some respite.

Stage 2: Hope with focused but big expenses. I think I might live longer than this. Let me spend on making my health better through supplements, therapies, yoga classes, and whatnot, so that I can live that time well, or even increase that time span. I can start saving once I am healthier.

Stage 3: Fear- or guilt-based reduction in expenses. I think I am certainly living longer than I had expected, but my health continues to deteriorate, so I might need money for future treatments and medication. I would need to save and invest. What if that is not enough?

Now I primarily oscillate between Stages 1 and 3, and my relationship with money changes accordingly. Should I invest in radically expensive alternative treatments so that I live longer, or do I save that money so that when I am dying, I do so with dignity? But what is dying with dignity, when there is no living with dignity? Should I release all stress or should I get those shoes that might reduce the pain when I walk? But what about the protein bar with all the right omegas or the organic anti-cancer everything that I must consume? Do I really need another doppler test, yet again? But what if there actually is something as the nth specialist fears? Should I work and lose the time that I could have spent on recovering? Am I earning right now so that I can save to earn time and regain the health I have already lost long ago?

Though I am aware of my mortality, I haven't achieved those acclaimed heights of wisdom or sainthood. I exist in the strangest of conflicts that I never thought I would face. My struggle is that I don't know my spending capacity and priorities because we don't know the future course of the illness and I have no insurance backup. Hence, no financial safety net. However, if you imagine I must now not be spending any money on pleasure, you couldn't be further from the truth! Should I be ashamed of my desires? I truly am. I mostly exist in trepidation or guilt. Contrary to hopes of surpassing lowly vanities and paradoxes, worrying does not provide clarity; it just makes things messier. At times a part of me even wants to fight against capitalism, for the algorithms that capitalize on my fears and desires, hounding me online for the turmeric with ten times more curcumin and the dress that will make me look desirable despite the illness tag. To fight the giants who make treatments cruelly inaccessible to those who need them desperately. Those are bigger battles, our collective battles; I am currently a tired mind in a tired body. I must begin the fight for my insurance and rights. I hope that when I fight, I fight for everyone else who might be struggling with the same.

I have shared my vulnerability with you unabashedly because I believe that fair insurance support could have relieved me of this undue madness. Don't ask me to meditate, join me in asking for a systemic change instead. I come from a relatively privileged background, and fortunately, my friends have access to networks and could ensure that the funds for my surgeries and chemotherapy were raised for me. Yet I am still finding it genuinely hard to cope with my altered life. Every day there are innumerable fundraiser videos circulating on the internet, how many of those patients receive their lifesaving injections or surgeries? I am distraught at the enormity of financial debts and strains, apart from the emotional and physical stress that these patients and their caregivers have to bear. I am much slower at work today than I was in 2018. I do not take up assignments with a lot of travel. I have to be ultra-careful with my food and hygiene. All of these reduces my options for work greatly. What happens to people who are not generalists like me? How do they find work if they cannot use their core skills anymore and are still recovering from illness? What if they are the sole earning members, what happens to their families? Will my elderly parents too continue to live with financial fears and restrictions because of my recurring expenses? The problem is not just insurance. It is the insanity of medical costs, the maze of these processes, that I alone won't be able to ever navigate, afford, or fight. At some point in our lives, each one of us might face this cruel reality, in one form or another. Yet, we do not ask for change. Why?

Cancer treatment has a lot of side effects, and one of the many challenging ones is starting afresh with financial vulnerability. If coupled with familial turbulence, relations under intense strain and fatigue, and uncommon complexities, it leaves you stranded. I am still coming to terms with it, four years later. I haven't yet figured out the right way to live, particularly financially, post my cancer diagnosis. I have found it hard to be present, to enjoy a moment as being enough. It has caused me to hurt the people I love the most for I have failed to respond to their constraints and their own lives' complexities with the compassion and understanding they deserve. It took me a while to realize that the root cause is not cancer alone but the lack of stability caused by the enormous financial implications that are a part of it. My greatest fear is that these battles will take away my tenderness. Will I be able to pause and experience gratitude? Will I be able to serve others if I'm obsessed with saving myself? Will there be solutions in collective care or mutual care that would ease these anxieties? Will I once again find the courage to carve my own unique path? I do not know.

I apologize for the rather dark image I must have painted; my intent is not to cause despair. My intent is to create through words a space for my agony and yours to be acknowledged. I am not offering refuge from pain. It is only after accepting the truth of our existence that we can take appropriate steps. I am leading myself to Stage 4 that's filled with acceptance and sadness. I want to be calm and fight with the grace that comes with knowing. This reflection is part of my process.

May you still be tender, may you stay courageous.

—Poornima Sardana

TREATMENTS:
AN INVESTMENT OR
EXPENSE?

"The FNAC is clean, don't worry!" the nurse reassured me with a smile.

I came back home much relieved. I had felt a lump in my right breast while going to bed one night. Within two days, I booked an appointment with the nearest gynecologist I found on Google. Without informing anyone at home, I went to see her. She looked worried after the examination and suggested that I get a mammography, an ultrasound, and a Fine Needle Aspiration Cytology (FNAC) done. This heightened my anxiety. I came back home dismayed. I disclosed the news to my parents, and they were equally disturbed. The next two days before the appointment were long and worrisome. Meanwhile, I was serving my notice period at the office since my family was supposed to immigrate to a new country within two months. A lot of things were happening simultaneously.

Mammography was excruciatingly painful, raising my doubts. The FNAC was horrific. I was so scared of even visiting the doctors because these tests caused a lot of mental stress that multiplied my physical pain! The reports suggested that I had a benign lump, so I went back to the doctor relieved. However, she suggested that we go for surgery soon. Something wasn't adding up. Deep inside,

I knew that I needed a second opinion. I visited gynecologist #2 who was recommended to me by a family member. This doctor was a blunt man who was enraged at seeing me visit a gynecologist for checking my breasts. "What are breast surgeons for?" he asked me furiously. I was so confused. To my knowledge, a gynecologist knew female anatomy best. Even in his exasperation, gynecologist #2 recommended a surgeon in North Delhi.

The situation didn't worry me anymore—the lump was benign—so I went to see this surgeon casually after a few weeks. He examined me and said that the lump felt bigger than what the report suggested and asked me to get the surgery done immediately. He was a general surgeon and said extracting a benign lump was the easiest operation he could conduct.

I was left with no choice but to get it done since my ticket to move to a new country was booked for the next month. I didn't have any time to waste.

Lying all scared on the stretcher, I was being wheeled into the operation theater in a local private hospital. I think the junior doctor saw me crying while praying. He asked me to calm down before giving me anesthesia. I woke up in the patients' ward with my mother by my side. I couldn't feel any pain, but I did feel light-headed. "The worst is over," I said to myself. I reassured my mother that I was doing fine and was discharged soon.

Who knew that the biopsy report of the lump would declare it malignant! When the doctor disclosed this news to me, the utter shock of hearing this news made me go numb. I asked him plainly, "What does it mean? What should be my next course of action?" He started saying words like completion surgery, cancer, and chemotherapy, which didn't make any sense to me. My parents were crying, but I was still unable to comprehend anything. "Did you say I have cancer? My report doesn't say anything like that!" He then explained how I had a very rare occurrence of an invasive papillary carcinoma in my right breast, which is an aggressive form of cancer.

To this my next question was, "But, I have already left my job to immigrate to a new country, do I have to turn back now?" He asked me to go see an oncologist for more insights.

Here started my ordeal of choosing doctors, hospitals, and treatments while I didn't even know how to swallow the news of carrying a deadly disease in my body. I was young and naïve when I learned about my condition, and I was clueless about how and which doctors to approach. The story unfolded so quickly that I couldn't even be a good enough audience to absorb it.

The sheer shock of learning that a lump thought to be benign can be malignant created doubts in our minds regarding the credibility of the highly acclaimed diagnostic center. I started looking for answers on Google. Yes, it was highly likely that a rare cancer like mine could go undetected in the fine needle test. The next step was to understand the medical establishments and how to find the right doctors. In our heads, cancer is a term that has a monolithic image. We just cannot imagine how wide its horizon is and how differently it plays out for each affected individual.

We were oscillating between different suggestions—government establishments, semi-private, and private institutions. With no job and only some savings for the future, I was really scared of the expenses lined up ahead. I had already borne an expense of about one lakh rupees to get my basic tests, doctor visits, and initial surgery done. I began to prepare myself for the next leg of treatment that was supposed to be elaborate and overwhelming, both financially and emotionally.

I had no insurance cover except for the one provided to me by my employer, but I was no longer eligible for it. The mammoth cost of the treatment was my real apprehension now, even more than my recovery. It was estimated to be around 25 lakh rupees. The savings from a decade of service in the corporate sector was supposed to support me in the future. Here I was signing up for a treatment that would wipe it off completely. It would not only punch a huge hole in my funds but also take a substantial chunk of my mother's retirement funds.

Medical facilities are difficult to navigate. I was totally lost between the advice I was getting from all directions about which hospital, doctor, and treatment was best for me. No one around me seemed to understand that every cancer is different and that there is no standardized treatment for all patients. I came to this understanding only after extensive research on the internet. I was so overwhelmed with the information online and offline (read unwarranted suggestions and future projections from anyone and everyone) at this point that I completely shut myself off.

Following my gut, I went to the breast onco-surgeon suggested to me by my first surgeon. She was associated with a very expensive private hospital and the establishment was intimidating. But as soon as I entered her room and spoke to her, I calmed down. She explained the course of the treatment to me and told me that I could conserve my affected breast. The suggested treatment included completion lumpectomy, in which the remaining breast tissue was to be removed. A sentinel lymph node biopsy was to be done to check if the cancer had spread further to the lymph nodes, followed by chemotherapy and radiotherapy to curb any cancerous growth in the body. But before all of this, I was subjected to a PET Scan.

The report suggested that the cancer had not spread anywhere in the body except for the site it was found at. Even this encouraging report didn't stop my doctor from slowing down.

She allowed me to go for my PR landing in Canada, as this was an important step for securing my future. But everything comes at a cost. We paid a huge amount to book last-minute two-way tickets for a soft landing and start our PR process. I came back to India within a week, to begin my treatment.

Without any mental or physical preparation, I was admitted to the hospital and thus began my treatment. The completion surgery was intensely painful. I had not anticipated the agony. While I was recovering from it, I was told about embryo freezing (cryopreservation) and how it was essential for a young woman like me to preserve my chances of being a mother in the future. We decided to go for it. Another expensive affair, but I wanted to secure my chances at motherhood. The process involved injections and everyday hospital visits, which meant more miscellaneous charges. This increased my expense by over 1.5 lakh rupees, while the completion surgery cost around one lakh rupees.

I was now heading for my medical treatment. The team of doctors taking care of my case decided that I should get 16 weekly cycles of chemotherapy. The first four were fortnightly and the last twelve were weekly. But before all of that, I had to undergo another surgical procedure to get a catheter (PICC line) inserted in my arm. It cost us about another lakh.

It was also mandatory to stay at the hospital after the first chemotherapy session for observation in case of any adverse reactions. We booked a room along with other amenities. The first chemotherapy session alone costed a whopping 50 thousand rupees.

For each session, I had to book a chemotherapy ward/room and take the medicines, food, and nursing services. Each session cost us about 25 thousand rupees. Only one-third of the cost of each session included the price of the medicine used. The rest was hospital overheads. I was lucky enough to be able to afford the exorbitant price at which this treatment was offered. I often wondered about the many patients who do not have the resources and how they would manage their disease.

The period of chemotherapy was long and painful. The COVID-19 pandemic made it worse. We were stepping out during lockdowns for my chemotherapy sessions. There was practically no one outside my immediate family that I could meet at that time. This took a toll on my mental health, and I even took the help of psychotherapy and meditation. By the time chemotherapy was over, most of my funds had been flushed. I was yet to undergo radiotherapy, a mandatory step in breast conservation surgeries. I was subjected to 20 cycles. With every cycle, the affected area became darker and more sensitive. Finally, after six months, when the treatment was over, I had borne a damage of about Rs 25 lakhs. But I thought that I would now be free and start my life again.

During my last visit to the doctor, she said, "You have recovered well, but we need to keep you under constant surveillance. Breast cancers tend to return, so we must be vigilant." I was stunned! Didn't I sign up for the treatment to be disease free? She said, "You are cancer free but in remission."

In the next three months, when my body was supposed to recover, I learned that my bones, ovaries, and liver had been adversely impacted by the chemotherapy and I needed further medication and injections to bring them back to normal. So, additional treatment was deployed to fight the side effects of the primary treatment. This time, the expense was borne completely by my family because I was out of funds. Even the miscellaneous treatment cost us over one lakh rupees.

Two years since then, I have moved countries, changed jobs, and earned back my expenditure on the treatment (which was between Rs. 25 and 30 Lakhs), but the nightmare still haunts me. Often, I wonder how much is too much? Is there any amount of money that secures us completely? Can there ever be decent medical facilities that cover treatments for critical illnesses? How would people qualify for such facilities—can we say no to someone? Everyone is fighting a battle we don't know about. Is there really a solution to it?

I am not sure if medical insurance is an answer to this problem because I know most people struggle with plans and claims. For patients like me who are young and in remission, getting insurance is a Herculean task. Firstly, no one is ready to offer one, and if someone does show interest, the premium is insane. I have been offered some weird plans offering coverage up to 2 lakhs for 2 years after which I can buy the insurance if I pay a sum of 10 lakhs in the next 5 years. Isn't that completely absurd? Does it even make sense to get myself insured with these ill-planned packages?

Rebuilding my life bit by bit, I often sit down and wonder whether these tools of medical insurance and reimbursements are designed to help those in need or are they just a means of earning profits? Are our treatments really an investment or an endless expenditure?

—Vani Verma

THE HARDEST DECISION
OF MY LIFE

The Beginning of the Recent Past

"Where do you see yourself in five years?"

Growing up I was asked this question a lot. Recently, when I tried to remember what I had wanted from life back then, all I could think of was what others had hoped from me. My parents were certain I would be married by now, my friends had hoped I would be dating someone decent, and my co-workers had assumed I would advance professionally.

But what had I wanted? I just couldn't recall. Frustrated, I decided to let it go. As I stood waiting in the billing queue, I wondered what had triggered such a thought at this time. With so much to worry about, why was I even thinking about that? It wouldn't matter anyway, for I certainly hadn't seen myself in the situation I ended up in. So, gathering my thoughts, I got my billing done and was informed it would be an hour before they called me in. Experience, however, had taught me that it would take much longer. As I handed my reports, I looked around the waiting room. This place was always crowded, with attendants running around and children and the elderly alike queuing for their turn. People were always complaining about the long waiting time for a few minutes of consultation, and I was always one of them. Today, however, I was in no hurry. I was dreading the conversation I was going to have with the doctor and wanted to put it off for as long as possible. I was so nervous that I felt I needed to calm myself before my turn. So, having found a seat at the far end, I plugged in my earphones and as I drowned out the voices around me, I couldn't help but reflect on the journey that had brought me to this point.

The Dreadful Diagnosis

It feels like it was only yesterday but at the same time also a lifetime ago. It was a typical weekday, like any other, till I felt a lump in my breast. My first thought was to wonder if it had always been there and if I had simply overlooked it. However, a casual mention of it to my mother sent her into a panic. She calmed down after I promised to go see a doctor. I wasn't really worried and the doctor's visit confirmed it. I was simply given a few supplements to take and I didn't make much of it. I was in my mid-20s, in the best shape of my life, had no known family history of cancer, ate well, exercised regularly, didn't smoke, and was in general particular about fitness. So, you would think I would be healthy, right? But then why was the lump still there even after six months? It even appeared to have grown in size. So, this time we decided to visit an oncologist. Not one, but two separate doctors assured us that everything was normal. These kinds of lumps were apparently common in women my age. And yet, something didn't feel right. It was probably my concerned expression that prompted the doctor to suggest a biopsy while maintaining that it was completely unnecessary.

Normally you would never see me in a lab unless a doctor absolutely and positively said I needed a test. But here I was, despite not even knowing what a biopsy entailed, insisting on getting one. So, after much persistence, and mostly for our peace of mind, my biopsy was scheduled. While I wasn't sure what to expect, as I held the report on my phone, I knew for certain that this was not what anyone had even wildly imagined—metastatic breast cancer!

Absorbing the Shock

With my diagnoses of stage IV cancer that had spread to the liver, hospitals quickly became my second home. The visits after my diagnosis, however, were very different from the ones before. Everything was happening too fast for us to process. Suddenly, this sense of urgency surrounded us, and it didn't give us a chance to think through what we were being told. We were all in shock and agreed to whatever protocol was suggested. I had to get a series of tests before the actual treatment. They included multiple MRIs, X-rays, scans, and of course blood tests. I was in and out of the hospital so much that I felt like a patient even before the treatment began. Through all this, my parents were shattered, and my friends were in shock. My response, however, was the most surprising of all.

One would assume I'd be devastated and crying uncontrollably for days in a situation like this. But I had barely cried. Looking back, I'm not sure I fully grasped the gravity of the situation. I was sad, but it was because of how things would change for me rather than the disease itself. Call it my defense mechanism, but I wasn't really feeling emotional at all. I was just going around behaving like cancer wasn't a big deal. I wasn't asking, "why me?" to assign blame, but to figure out what I could do. I was only interested in learning what went wrong and finding answers. And I wasn't getting any satisfactory ones. For example, after consulting with a geneticist, we discovered that my cancer wasn't genetic. We were told that it's a lifestyle disease and many people nowadays have cancer that is not genetic. So, naturally, I wanted to know what changes I needed to make in my lifestyle to combat it. But none were suggested. Instead, I was told to keep living the way I did and just have chemo, and everything would be fine. Sure, they gave a few do's and don'ts to follow while undergoing the treatment, but no overall lifestyle changes were suggested. I had hoped to try alternative treatments alongside the allopathic one but was advised not to. My doctors insisted that tracking the effectiveness of treatments would be difficult if a variety of medications were involved. I wasn't against chemo in any way, but it would have been nice to hear another point of view. But, despite my reservations, knowing that dealing with the tumor was the top priority, I agreed to the protocol and we began my chemo.

Chemo Is No Therapy

I was very nervous about my first chemo session because I had only heard negative things about it. This was obviously heightened by all the articles I read online. So, I was surprised to find the actual process to be relatively simple. You don't have to do much. You are simply connected to an IV drip and can relax while the medications take effect. The tricky part, however, starts when the side effects start kicking in. While there is a list of expected reactions, there is no way to predict how a patient will react. While some exhibit symptoms in addition to the expected ones, others show no symptoms at all. You also never know when these effects will appear. You could be fine after one cycle and extremely ill after the next one.

A few weeks in and even I began to exhibit the common and expected side effects. It started with minor joint pains and a puffy face from the steroids. Then, my hair started falling, slowly but steadily. Soon my periods stopped, my nails were discolored, and I was almost completely bald in a matter of months. Fortunately, unlike many others, I didn't experience severe symptoms, either because of my age or because of my general overall health.

The first scan after my treatment showed a really good response. This was interpreted positively by doctors, so much so that a family doctor suggested, to my bewilderment, that we consider not stopping my chemo at all. He reasoned that because my cancer was so aggressive, and I was responding well to the treatment, this could be our way to delay relapse. Thankfully, a few cycles later, my reports were what doctors considered stable, and the doctors in charge of my treatment decided to discontinue the chemo. I was still required to continue with the maintenance. They specified no timeline as to how long I'll have to continue with it, but I was too happy to be off chemo to complain.

Soon, I went from visiting the hospital once every few days to once every few weeks and I considered this to be a significant improvement. Gradually, we started getting into a routine. With time, my hair had started growing back (this time curly), my periods were back (which I took as a really good sign of recovery), and I was soon stepping out without a wig. Call me crazy, but among all of these, I was happiest the day I thought my eyebrows had grown back sufficiently enough to be shaped once more. Who would have imagined how satisfying getting your eyebrows threaded could be after such a long time! Everything seemed to be slowly getting back to normal. Health-wise too, things appeared to be stabilizing, or so we thought.

Cancer Really Is Like a Crab

Coincidentally, one year later around the same time as my first scan, we were back in the hospital, with another scan showing an increase in the tumor. We all just froze on seeing the report. I just couldn't think straight. What did this mean for me? The prospect of going through chemo once again was almost unfathomable. When we met the doctors, we learnt that since the tumor hadn't spread much, they were debating the suitable protocol. Seizing the opportunity, I literally begged them not to restart the chemo. After a little deliberation, they agreed and instead gave me oral medications for the time being while continuing the maintenance. These medications had their own set of side effects, but I was too relieved to be bothered. What we didn't realize then, however, was that this incident was just the beginning of a pattern in my treatment that would continue.

The medicines worked and the scans were stable in a few months and we rejoiced. But it only lasted for a short while. A few months later, another scan revealed a slight growth, and the medications were changed again. I was told that this was the nature of the disease. It would continue to mutate, and they would keep changing the medications and dosages to keep it under control. In short, I had to stay in treatment forever. The word "stable" lost its significance. While a negative scan caused panic, stable scans only meant continuing the treatment. There was no end in sight.

Lifespan versus Quality of Life

While everyone was focusing on increasing my lifespan, it seemed as if they were ignoring how this affected the quality of my life. I was confined mostly to home and hospital. Making any kind of spontaneous plans was out of the question. I had to meticulously plan everything around my hospital schedule, and now even that appeared impossible. Any second a new development could change everything. My queries about how long we could keep this up were met with responses like, "As long as your body can handle it." To me it essentially indicated that they would keep continuing till all was fine, knowing well that these medicines inherently had the potential to cause major side effects over time. In case of a major side effect, like organ failure, they would cease the treatment to concentrate on fixing that problem instead. While I was aware of the risks from the beginning, I had naively believed that the treatments would end in a few months.

I didn't anticipate they would keep upping the medications after each scan, and I certainly didn't anticipate to be in treatment indefinitely.

This was when I started looking out for support groups in the hope to meet someone who could empathize. Over the years, I had the opportunity to meet many patients of various ages. I was even introduced to a few young survivors. While it was nice to connect with someone my age who had gone through something similar, I realized I had less in common with them than I thought. Everyone seemed to have a different treatment and associated set of problems.

For example, one survivor, who is now a good friend, was diagnosed at an early stage. As a result, she had only needed an operation. No chemo or radiation. So, while we sympathized with each other, we couldn't relate to each other's journeys. Even among this large group of cancer survivors, I was alone, looking for a support group that didn't exist. It was all very tiring.

Real Advocacy Begins amidst Unreal Circumstances

Cancer is probably the only disease in which a patient can walk in looking healthy and come out of the treatment totally broken. I was close to giving up on the treatment many times but each time was talked back into continuing. That was until one scan a few cycles ago. My tumor grew again, as was the pattern, but this time the doctors suggested surgery. I was told very early on in my diagnosis that because it was metastatic, surgery would have little effect and there would still be a very high chance of recurrence. So, the suggestion at this point surprised me. When I asked if the chances of recovery from surgery had improved, the answer was still negative.

I didn't want to be cut open for something with low chances of success. It would have been different if the doctors were confident that this was the right path to take. But here, it was more like, "We've tried everything, why not try this approach?" I failed to see what I would gain from this ordeal. So, I decided to say no to the surgery. The doctors were not pleased and advised me to reconsider. Perhaps it wasn't the best decision, but I was done. I was done with this trial-and-error approach. I was done getting these treatments forever. Done waiting for scans to show growth and changing my treatment again.

I had wanted to try alternative treatments before and decided it was time I gave it a shot. I knew I couldn't leave then because my scans were all over the place. So, I agreed to the alternative protocol for the time being. That also meant I would have time to convince everyone. Getting my family to understand why I was taking this decision was going to be a challenge. My sister was the easiest to get on board. She understood that it was not practical to ask me to continue like this forever. My parents, however, were not even willing to talk about it. Every time I brought it up, they would change the subject. If I pushed, it would turn into an argument, so I gave up. I reasoned to myself that I could talk to the doctors first and get them on board by explaining my need for a break, and perhaps they could assist me in explaining the decision to my parents. I spent my entire time coming up with arguments I would present to the doctors. I felt like I was back in law school preparing for a moot court competition, except this was about my life.

I kept making and arguing my case in my head over the months trying to convince myself more than others that this was the right call. Never had I waited in anticipation for anything as I did my next scan. Finally, it was time. All I hoped for was that the reports were stable.

The Dissenters Were My Well-wishers

I took in a deep breath as I opened my eyes. There was still a long queue of impatient patients around me. I pulled out my report from the bag, just to recheck. Yes, I was stable! I could finally have the discussion about stopping my treatment, at least temporarily! I had purposefully come to the hospital alone. I was expecting the doctors to try to talk me out of it and I didn't want them to use emotions to persuade my parents. I kept going over the arguments I had prepared over these past months as I waited. Soon they called my name. The nurse told me to hurry because the doctor had to leave for a meeting after my turn. Seeing the report, the doctor was happy. We could continue with the protocol. She was smiling at me when I suddenly just blurted it out, "I want to stop the treatment." I wanted to say more but I seemed to be at a loss for words. I just kept staring at her. The smile had disappeared. She quietly wrote something on her sheet, grabbed her phone, and left—probably for her meeting. Her junior just handed me my reports as I kept wondering if the doctor was coming back.

I was in shock at what just transpired. So that was it. Was it *this* easy to stop the treatment? It all seemed quite anticlimactic in hindsight. As I left, I couldn't help but wonder why I wasn't feeling relieved. Wasn't this what I had wanted? It was the doctor's indifference that somehow hurt me the most. One would think that after all these years, the doctor would be slightly more invested. While I was clear about my decision, I was at least hoping they would want to talk about it, maybe ask me about my alternative plans, anything. Instead, they simply let me go. It was like the second I disagreed, I no longer mattered. Slightly put off by this, I reached home. While my big announcement at the hospital didn't go as planned, it received the expected reaction at home. Tears, anger, accusations, and, of course, prayers. My parents even called my friends, relatives, and anyone else they thought could persuade me. But I kept explaining my point to everyone. They even suspected I was suicidal for not wanting to continue with the treatment. Deep down though, I think they were aware that the treatment was not a cure, only palliative care, but in the absence of a cure, it was better than nothing. And I totally understood their pain. I had taken the decision because I was tired, but viewing from the lens of a parent, I could see how hard it was for them. I have to give them the credit for they gradually did come around. I am certain that it has not been easy for them to sit and watch, not knowing when I can suddenly take a turn for the worse. They have been more supportive than I had ever imagined and I feel that I need to be fine for their sake now more than mine.

To Be Continued. Hopefully

I still can't remember what I thought I would be when I grew up, but this is where I am now: a 30-year-old metastatic cancer patient who has stopped her treatment in search of alternative cures. There is no moral or great conclusion to this story. I don't know what I have gained from all this or where it will lead me. All I tell myself is that back in the hospital the doctors were experimenting on me and now I am doing that to myself. I am still looking out for alternatives that might work for me, and when I recover, I hope to document this crazy second half of my journey in detail. I don't blame the doctors. I know that they were doing their best. It is just that their approach didn't seem right for my condition. So, while I don't regret giving alternative treatment a chance over allopathy, when I look back, I do wish I didn't have to pick one over the other. As I continue on the path I chose, I do hope in the future all forms of medicine work in harmony, instead of competing with one another because only when a patient benefits from the wisdom of all fields can we truly achieve holistic healing.

—Pallavi Saraswatula

FOLLOWING CAREGIVERS' JOURNEYS

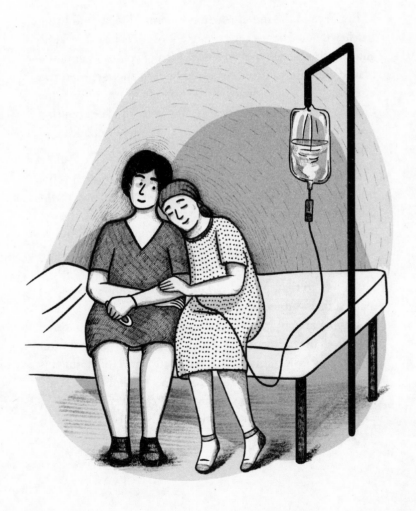

Imagine finding out your loved one has cancer. You might feel like the wind got knocked out of your lungs. You are left gasping for air. Your eyes turn into a broken dam and the tears can't be stopped. Or you might go completely numb, not registering what's happening. You might even ignore what's happening or be in denial. All of these are common and acceptable reactions. Everyone deals with the diagnosis in their own way as a caregiver.

But beyond the initial reaction is a long, lonely, and tiring journey that a caregiver must embark on. It is heartbreaking, gut-wrenching, and soul-crushing, forcing you to maintain a brave facade in front of your loved one. As the caregiver, you often end up suspending your own needs to prioritize being there for the one you're caring for. But you can't keep pouring from an empty cup, so you have to find ways to take care of yourself as well.

There might come a time to have uncomfortable conversations about end-of-life care and how your loved one might want to be treated if they can't communicate on their own. You might avoid having these conversations, lest it seem like you have given up all hopes and are hastening their death. However, asking them in advance and respecting their wishes, if it comes to that, might help in their final hours instead of making them suffer because you can't let them go. In spite of everything and all your efforts, you might also end up losing your loved one to the illness. How do you move forward from the pain of losing them? Can you really move on from this grief and loss or do you grow around it? Find out how some of our co-authors who are or have been caregivers are dealing with grief and pain and have their own ways of coping with the care or loss of a loved one.

MY OWN DANNY DENZONGPA

Every year, a few days before April 15, my parents and I have an intense discussion which bears no fruit. It is about what to get Meher, my brother, for his birthday. What can one get a man who supposedly has everything? Or the money to buy everything that we could buy for him. It also doesn't help that none of us understand the things he is passionate about—mostly some form of technology. We're pretty vanilla tech users. For example, while cooking, the most advanced appliance I use is a mixer-grinder or an oven. He likes to experiment with a sous vide machine—an appliance whose name I don't even know how to pronounce, let alone know how to use it.

I don't recall the exact conversation that happened on the eve of 15th last year, but I'd like to believe it was some version of the same discussion. Since I eat dinner earlier than my parents, I was just hanging around, giving them company while they had their late dinner. There is an unsaid rule of not bringing phones to the table and using this time for catching up instead. So, it was surprising that my mother left the table in a hurry saying something about getting calls repeatedly. My father and I discovered later that both of us also had missed calls from my sister-in-law, Kiran.

Kiran asked my mother to include everyone in the call. I took the phone from her and set it against some utensil. My father came and stood beside me on the left and my mother on the right. The only time I'd seen Kiran cry was at her *bidai*, so it was worrisome to see her teary-eyed. She shared that Meher had been feeling unwell the last couple of days and the diagnosis was serious.

He'd had COVID-19 in January 2021 while on a work visit to Dubai. Although that was a tense time for everyone, we'd gotten over that with relative ease compared to what many families in India and the world had to go through. Yes, Meher did have some fatigue even after recovering. But with the casual, unscientific reasoning so typical to most of us, we had attributed the fatigue and sickly look to the lasting impact of COVID-19.

Kiran and Meher had moved to Basel, Switzerland, in early March. They were in the process of settling down—finding a nanny for their two-and-a-half-year-old son Zubin, setting up a new home, and looking for a new job for Kiran. Although it was their second stint in the city, they had to adjust anew to the country, especially as young parents. In the middle of this, my observant brother realized his resting heart rate was at 90 beats per minute. Since he'd been running regularly for over two decades, his normal resting heart rate was around 45 bpm. Elevated heart rate along with an episode of fainting prompted him to consult a doctor. The doctor dismissed him as a hypochondriac, he later told me. Who goes in for a consultation claiming just an elevated resting heart rate as a cause for concern? Nonetheless, some blood tests were done and alas! My brother was diagnosed with Acute Lymphoblastic Leukemia (ALL). Acute implies a fast-spreading disease and leukemia is commonly known as blood cancer.

So, when Kiran said Meher has been diagnosed with leukemia, my father became eerily quiet. He had recently recovered from a life-threatening disease himself during which he'd lost the capacity to walk for over a month. However, he had bounced back with his typical indomitable spirit. My mother didn't understand the diagnosis too well. She assumed it was some eating-related disorder because Meher had been following intermittent fasting for a year and had lost a lot of fat. I guess it's a typical Indian mother's reaction to assume everything wrong with her child is because they are not eating "well." When she started grumbling about his fasting, I had to pause and confirm with Kiran if by leukemia she meant blood cancer. Because these diseases only happen in movies, don't they? The only person I'd heard of having blood cancer was Danny Denzongpa in China Gate—a movie I'd possibly seen along with my brother as a child. Danny's character was a Stage 4 blood cancer patient running around, climbing mountains, killing bandits, and saving children. I would often tease my brother that that's the ideal he should aim for and we'd have a good laugh. I discovered that both of us, my brother and I, have a dark sense of humor and it felt good to find something in common even when we were struggling.

I do not recall the rest of the conversation with Kiran. I assume it was full of logistical details about what the next steps were, where would the treatment take place, and how would COVID-19 impact his treatment. I would discover over the course of the treatment that we, as a family, were excellent at discussing the mundane and brushing aside the emotional.

Once I was alone in my room, I spoke to my partner, Swapnil. He was going through one of the darkest periods of his life—his father was a cancer patient undergoing chemotherapy, and he had had to put his doctoral studies on hold to support his family. When I scrolled back to the texts I sent him on that particular evening, I noticed one thing I repeated twice in a span of twenty texts. It seemed my brother had called me the same morning, before he'd received news of his diagnosis. I was in the middle of my workday so I hadn't looked away from my screen and had probably spoken to him in a distracted manner. Later, I was consumed by the possibility that that was the "last" call my brother made to me and I didn't even give him my full attention. There was a sense of finality I attached to his diagnosis. My naivety makes me smile now—in most cases, diagnosis is only the start of a journey of finding a path back to normalcy. And needless to say, the journey itself is harder than the beginning.

The next morning, I emailed my managers informing them of the diagnosis and setting up a call to discuss the possibility of a long absence. I thought that I would need their support the most in balancing my career and supporting my brother through his illness. Many colleagues have since expressed surprise and appreciation at my choosing to take a sabbatical of three months to support my brother and putting my career "on hold." Honestly, it was never a decision that I made consciously after weighing the pros and cons. To me, the fact that my brother came first was self-evident. I was not blind to the risks of such a decision. A long absence means effectively highlighting to your team and seniors that you're replaceable. It can affect promotions, bonuses, and growth besides a long gap, which is hard to return from under any circumstances. However, I was confident that I would find another job if I had to let go of this one. Maybe it wouldn't be equally good, but careers rarely have a linear path and I would find my way eventually. I certainly was not going to find another brother. Two of us came in a package—like the imli candies wrapped in plastic—and I was committed to doing whatever I could to keep the other candy intact.

Now, all of this was unfolding during the peak of the second wave of COVID-19 cases in India. International travel was restricted. We had to navigate through a maze of COVID-19-related administrative barriers. For instance, the Swiss embassy was issuing visas only for exceptional cases (for which we obviously qualified given the serious medical diagnosis), but one had to make a journey to Delhi as local visa facilitation centers were shut for business. Even I was fearful to undertake this journey, let alone my parents who are senior citizens. We kept pushing our plans to travel in the hope that the wave would subside. But our plans had to be moved forward when after a month of hospitalization my brother returned home and had an episode of delirium. The unpredictability of the disease, particularly the effects of the treatment, was a rude wakeup call. It was decided that my parents would visit for a month in July 2021 and I would stay from August to October 2021 for a period of 90 days—the maximum duration permitted on a visitor visa.

I also took time to understand that treatment schedules are rarely predictable. Modern medicine does indeed have clear protocols, at least for the disease my brother had, but every patient is different. There is only so much certainty one can expect. In the first month after the diagnosis, I would often get mildly irritated at how many times plans would change. With a treatment plan of eight intensive months followed by two years of at-home care, it was only in the fourth or fifth month that I recall having a clear path of where we were headed. At one point, there was a possibility that a bone marrow transplant would be required if conventional chemotherapy failed to produce results. The obvious choice of a donor was me—being his sibling—but only if I was a 100% match. So, in the middle of figuring out visas, collecting visa documents for my parents, and getting vaccinated in a hurry because the 18-40 age group had just been allowed starting May 1, I was figuring out what human leukocyte antigen typing really means and how I can get it done sitting at home. Unfortunately, I was only a 50% match with my brother. Although bone marrow transplant was dropped from the treatment plan given how well my brother's body reacted to chemotherapy (he was in remission within 60 days and has continued to be so!), being a part match implies that a search would be undertaken for a perfect match, if the need ever arose.

The question that was frequently on my parents' mind after the diagnosis was why did my brother get cancer? Here was a strong, healthy, and successful child, who would probably be their support in their sunset years, now suddenly needing their support to pull through. I would often lose patience, especially with my mother, when she would try to reason through this question. It didn't seem pertinent to me. But I can now begin to empathize with the depth of their despair. During a conversation, someone pointed out to me that there is a term for someone who loses their parent(s)—an orphan—but we have no term in the English language for a parent who has lost their child. It is against the natural order of things. And perhaps for this reason, it was very important for my parents to have this question answered. There are, of course, no answers available yet. Science hasn't progressed enough to give causal answers, only correlations. Being religious, they spent a large part of their energy and time seeking solace in prayers and rituals. I still, however, see that this unexpected turn of events affected them more deeply than me. Every action is viewed from the lens of cancer and there is no break from it.

There is no doubt that after my brother, this is the hardest for my sister-in-law. Imagine a young couple who've done well in life. They have had successful careers, are growing their family, and planning for bigger things to come. A relatively smooth ride is then disrupted to such an extent that the new life doesn't resemble the old one at all. All the possible trajectories you'd foreseen change overnight. Not only are you coming to terms with the long-term implications of a diagnosis such as cancer, but you also have to rapidly figure out the day-to-day adjustments, all while keeping it together emotionally. It is exceptional how well my sister-in-law, Kiran, adapted to this new status quo. She quit her job and became a full-time caregiver to her son and her husband. Although Switzerland has superior healthcare and insurance, she deftly navigated through unfamiliar systems. She has organized their life down to the minutest details. My brother has been drinking boiled water given his weakened immune system. He needs to drink 3 liters of water daily. Now to ensure that he always has a supply of boiled water, Kiran experimented with electric kettles and insulated bottles. Finally, she settled on tea kettles to boil and store water. A minor detail, but speaks volumes about Kiran's tenacity to battle through tough times.

I had some idea of what to expect when I finally did get to Basel. I saw on video calls that my brother looked like a shadow of his former self—a tall, well-built body with a thick head of hair was replaced by a lanky frame, balding head, and sunken eyes. I knew I'd have to shoulder responsibilities at their home ranging from cooking, cleaning, and babysitting to shopping for groceries and accompanying my brother on hospital visits. I'd have to adjust to the new weather, new people, and a completely new language. I'd like to believe I did all of the above as adeptly as possible. What took me by surprise was the effort it took to constantly put myself second. I was physically and, more importantly, emotionally pushing myself harder than I ever had. It was like taking the hardest and most bizarre exam—you never signed up for it, there is no measure of success/failure, the stakes are high, because it is literally a matter of life or death, there are no lectures you can attend, and no teacher can guide you. Bear in mind that I was neither the patient nor the primary caregiver! I had the luxury of running the marathon from one check-post to another and then going back to being a spectator, cheering from the sidelines.

This year my parents and I engaged in that futile discussion of what to gift my brother for his birthday yet again. My brother and I discovered a common love for European cheese during our three months together. So, I did some research on how I could deliver some high-quality, organic cheese to his home. I shortlisted a few options and then abandoned the whole idea. I look forward to doing this year after year because every time I do this is yet another year my brother has lived cancer-free.

—Piuli Roy Chowdhury

EVERY DAY IS A NEW STORY

When I saw my brother for the first time after his diagnosis, I cried. It had already been three and a half months since we knew. He had had multiple rounds of stay at the hospital for his chemotherapy. We'd constantly been in touch—talking once, sometimes even twice a day, much higher than our usual frequency of twice a month. Despite the conversations, the preparations for the physical and metaphorical journeys and some expectations of what this phase would be like, I was overcome with emotion at seeing my brother.

I reached Basel, Switzerland, where my brother lived, on August 1, 2021. My brother was hospitalized for an ongoing round of chemotherapy and so we had to plan to go meet him during visitation hours. My sister-in-law, Kiran, along with my three-year-old nephew, Zubin, and I arrived at the hospital and waited in the garden for my brother to come see us. The garden at the university hospital is beautiful. It has large trees with benches underneath. A small pond with colorful fishes can be crossed by a tiny bridge. There is a play area for children with small slides and swings. Ironically, there is also a smoking enclosure which is usually the center of activity. I became well versed with the ins and outs of this garden because of the number of hours I spent giving company to my brother during his hospitalizations. But on the first day I visited him, I sat enjoying the weather and the scenery until I saw him.

I knew what he looked like in theory. He'd lost a lot of fat and muscle. Since his hair had started falling due to the side effects of chemo, he'd shaved it all off. My brother was known for his lustrous, black, and thick hair. We often called it the "Russian Hat." It was curiously spiky as a child (nicknamed porcupine then) and as he grew older it became more and more like the winter hat traditionally worn by Russians. No matter how he combed, it fell in the same unmanageable way. His eyes have this unexplained quality of changing color in the sunlight. It goes from dark brown to the color of honey. But now I barely noticed the color of his eyes as they had sunk deep into his skull with rings of dark circles underneath. And although it was a warm European summer evening, he was dressed in a jacket for even a minor cold could take days to get rid of, slowing down an already torturously long treatment plan of eight months. As he approached me, I hugged him and started tearing up. It's hard to explain why it's odd that something as minor as tears upon meeting is worth a mention. I come from a family where we don't express vulnerability as openly as we should. I felt embarrassed, concerned, and weak all at once. But I also felt normal. It felt good to hug him—as if it confirmed that he was still around and this was a battle we could win.

We settled into a rhythm quickly. If my brother was in the hospital, I would deliver food to him twice a day. The rest of the day would be spent planning and executing tasks for those two meals. I had some experience in the homely Indian cooking that most households do—the sabzi-roti-daal-chawal combination. We would supplement that with sandwiches, corn, and olives. On the days my brother was at home, he decided to pursue a new hobby—cooking. This was an eyebrow-raising choice because his starting point was laughably poor. If asked to boil milk, he'd probably not know which utensil to use. I could bet a ridiculous amount of money that he couldn't even differentiate between the spices most commonly used in Indian cooking. So armed only with his inexplicable confidence and zero knowledge, he immersed himself in the videos of Chef

Ranveer Brar online. It got so bad that I would walk into his room and he'd make a guilty face as if he was hiding something and it'd turn out to be a Ranveer Brar video. It would have been less embarrassing to have caught him watching pornography.

As he was learning a new hobby, I was also learning something about him. So far, the areas of life that he had excelled in were so alien to me that I was never able to place why exactly he was so good at the things he did. But in this case, it happened to be an activity in which I had some prior experience. The first thing I observed was that he never backed down from a challenge. He would pick up the harder recipes and see them through. We tried the railway cutlet—a favorite snack of those who've traveled by the Indian Railways. That recipe had so many elements in the preparation section itself that I would have never attempted it if I was cooking alone. The second was his appetite for taking risks. He loved experimenting and would often come up with wacky combinations like mango-chili flavored dhoklas—a steamed dish made from gram flour and yogurt. Or make a vegetable broth from scratch that took 3 hours of boiling for some Japanese Udon noodles that he finally declared were too far from the real thing and refused to eat! And finally, his ability to take critical feedback. He once negotiated with his doctors to come home for a few hours during his hospitalization to make tomato soup. I honestly didn't enjoy it and said as much, which he accepted graciously.

Hospital visits and cooking projects were also our time for conversations. We would mostly indulge in banter, but once in a while, we would talk about life and death. These are conversations you typically expect to have in your twilight years, right? But when faced with a potentially fatal and unpredictable disease, that process gets fast-forwarded and at the age of 33, you ask yourself whether you've lived a good life. What was the purpose of it all? What would death look like? Was your karma good enough? Possibly not for rebirth, but as a legacy for your children. I am open to uncomfortable conversations, and in this scenario, it turned out to be useful. Once the three of us, my brother, an elderly relative, and I were cooking together and he mentioned his death casually. This made our relative uncomfortable and she looked to me for support in asking my brother to not verbalize the unsaid. I had a different approach to conversations about his death. Of course, there is no question that death would be the worst outcome for all, but there was a large probability of surviving and figuring out a new status quo. I would acknowledge the former, but pull his focus toward the latter. I never expected my brother (or I for that matter) to stop thinking about his death, but I tried my best to think beyond his death as well.

With the scientific temper so natural to him, his appetite for unusual questions and even more bizarre answers, and an unbelievable risk-taking attitude, he seriously began to consider the possibility of cryonics. For a layperson, cryonics is a field of study that focuses on how to preserve the human body for eventual resurrection after clinical death if and when such technology becomes available. In short, humanity can freeze and preserve bodies, but has no tech to bring them back to life! I am sure every reader at this point has questions exploding in their mind like fireworks. Unfortunately, I am ill-equipped to answer any question scientifically, so I recommend a short detour to Google.

Since I found out about cryonics, I have asked many close ones if they'd ever sign up for it if they had the resources. I have heard a resounding no every single time. Imagine your lifeless body undergoing an alien procedure so far removed from the "normal" that the only movie I can reference as an example is Captain America who remains frozen for 60 years.

My brother and I would often joke that maybe blood cancer is really his path to becoming a superhuman and who knows cryonics may actually make it happen! Not only does he come back to life 400 years later, but there is technology available to genetically free him of the disease and make him indestructible! Woohoo!

Regarding the alien procedures, you can argue that you're dead so it hardly matters what happens to your body, right? Then comes the uncertainty of how long you're actually going to remain frozen. This is not significant while you're frozen, but if and when you're brought back to life. When will that be, if ever? 200 years later? 400? 1000? If we brought back a person from the 1970s, they'd probably not understand how to use a smartphone we take for granted today. What kind of society from a cultural, technological, political, and environmental perspective will you be confronted with after years of being frozen? How will society view these "zombies" and how will they be rehabilitated and integrated back into civilization? I can go on and on with these musings. The point is, despite so many "whys" and "whats" I understood the only "why" that really mattered—why it was important for my brother to sign up for this. His intense love for life overcame every fear about a future, even a future as wildly uncertain as this one. And when he mentioned it to me, I promised to support if there was any resistance to his wishes. The only thing that bothered me was that there would be nobody to bid goodbye to if it came to pass suddenly—today or 50 years later, but I guess it was a small cost to pay.

Contrary to my expectations, my family, especially my parents, were accepting of his decision to undergo cryopreservation. I had assumed the missed Hindu rites of passage would be a deterrent to their acceptance, but upon consideration I realized that contemplating a child's death is unnatural and they would rather avoid it. When my brother did contractually agree to cryopreservation, he explained the process and its significance. I honestly don't know how they felt about it. It is possible that they thought it was just another odd thing my brother had agreed to do and something they didn't expect to see in their lifetime.

However, the decision to cryopreserve wasn't made in a day. I suspect it was during the month-long hospitalization in September 2021 that my brother went from a maybe-let's-do-it to I-am-definitely-doing-this. His treatment had been ongoing since mid-April. Each hospitalization was followed by reaction to the therapy, faltering recovery, and then again, the downhill journey to the next round. In addition to chemical infusions, he was given spinal injections of chemo which were painful because they led to constant headaches for days after. Though he started chemotherapy with a relatively healthy body, by September he was probably at his worst and about to begin the hardest part of the treatment. During the first ten days of September the number of COVID-19 cases in Switzerland had gone down, so the doctors would allow him to visit home for a few hours if his test results were good. But after a while, that stopped completely, and he began feeling caged at the hospital. I would arrive equipped with a picnic mat, homemade food, extra warm clothes, and a backgammon board. We would find a new spot on the hospital grounds every day and lounge in the sunlight as long as he felt comfortable. It was a sunny month frequently complemented by a light breeze. As my brother slept on the picnic mat, I would read, walk around, or gaze blankly at my surroundings. The peaceful surroundings didn't reflect the tumultuous state of our minds. My brother, usually so put-together even in the face of this disease, suddenly spiraled into dark thoughts with questions like, "Do I have what it takes to get through?" As he battled his fears, so did the rest of us. I kept wondering if I was up to the task of being a sponge to his emotions, soaking it all in, but also squeezing it all out far away from him. By the end of the month, I was searching for flights back home and was on the verge of cutting short my three-month trip. It was one of my closest friends who acknowledged my pain since no one was aware of it. She helped me appreciate that uprooting my life in India and making Switzerland my temporary home was not easy. Just by being present, I was surely making a difference. I don't know how much I still believe in her words, but it worked at that point and I stayed.

It has been more than nine months since the intensive treatment ended and my brother was put on lower oral chemotherapy doses as maintenance treatment (expected to continue till December 2023). This phase is critical because the chances of a relapse are as high as

30% and will reduce dramatically once the medication is over. My brother has resumed his pre-cancer lifestyle in some measure. He works four to five hours a day, is allowed to eat a variety of foods, and can take short trips with precautions. Nonetheless, it is in many ways a "new normal." There are regular visits to the hospital, frequent medical scares like chicken pox, colds, COVID-19, and the looming question of what happens if there is a relapse—the fear of which is like your own shadow, following you everywhere, but you're just unaware of it. When you suddenly throw light on it, it becomes large and scary.

Someone undergoing a similar life experience recently said the following to me when I asked about her husband's health—*har roz ek nayi kahani hai* (every day is a new story). I think it is true for humanity in general, but especially so for those who are fighting a disease like cancer. Your cancer type will be different, circumstances in life will be different, and how you respond is surely different, but what is common is that you're living a new story every day. I tell myself to accept each story with grace and humility because any story is better than no story.

—Piuli Roy Chowdhury

REBEL GIRL SAMRIDDHI

Dear Reader,

This is perhaps a story one dreads to read, lest death become a reality for themselves or their dearest one. But in case you find yourself here, I want you to know that life does continue, one terrible day after another, even after the loss of the center of your universe. You continue to live, continue to breathe, bask in the warm glow of their memories, and hope to one day continue all the conversations when you are together on the other side. You seek solace in dreams, in the mystery of signs, and continue to find ways to care for and love them.

This chapter is written in loving memory of my sister, dearest Samriddhi, who braved cancer and decided to live and leave on her own terms.

Mirroring Samriddhi

"I can guarantee her cancer will come back like I can guarantee the sun will rise again tomorrow," a friend, who was also a medical doctor, had once explained to me in exasperation. For endless hours I had been speaking to him about how the chemo was shrinking her tumors, and how hopeful we were that my sister would be free of cancer soon. We knew she would be a miracle case; we were confident. And we had our reasons to believe:

- The oncologist had assured us that her young age meant she could tolerate stronger doses of chemotherapy
- The supplements we were making her take—Tibetan medicine, Ayurvedic medicine, ocean medicine, cow therapy medicine, (insert the name of any other herbal medicine under the sun), magical religious concoctions, and the healing gems—"gave her an edge"
- The astrologers and shamans we thronged all assured us of a very long, happy life
- And oh, we even chanted the Mrityunjay mantra 9999999999999999 times

My friend had lost his patience at my unwillingness to accept the truth and was hammering it in my head, "You need to have an honest conversation with your sister about her end-of-life care." But talking about it meant acknowledging that we may lose her to cancer. And that felt like I was making the prospect more real.

When we were young, Samriddhi and I loved playing a game inspired from *Sophie's Choice*. One of our favorite questions was— would you rather die suddenly in an accident or slowly with an illness? She would often choose "slowly with an illness." Her reason was that it would give the family the time to expect, process, and prepare for the loss. Little did we know that death, no matter what the scenario, is unimaginably painful.

My sister lived through breast cancer and then again through brain cancer. However, when it's your own family, it is impossible to expect, process, or prepare for the fact that you might lose them one day. No matter what, you believe you will pull through, even when the doctors slap you with reality.

With extreme reluctance, I heeded my friend's request and decided to bring up the topic with my sister. We sat on the roof of our apartment building, dangling our legs on the edge, soaking in the sun, and staring into the eyes of the distant Boudhanath Stupa.

"Samriddhi, what if, and I'm only being hypothetical... your treatment is going so well right now and I'm certain it will work this time, but what if, like in a very tiny 0.00001 percent hypothetical scenario, what if the treatment gets difficult? Do you want to talk about what the options for care are at that stage?" I blurted out, throttled by the weight of the conversation. Feeling like I had made death a plausible reality by articulating the words, I wished for the conversation to end even before it began.

"Oh my god! I have been wanting to talk about this for SO long. I know Avi (her husband) can't handle these conversations and I wasn't sure whom to speak to. I'm so glad you brought this up," she said with what seemed like relief.

What does end-of-life care even mean? We discussed if a ventilator would be an option. She said yes sure, if there are chances of survival, you can try out a ventilator for a week. Thanks to Hindi movies, in our heads, a ventilator felt like an incubator where one would peacefully stick their head in for however long it was needed. Second on the list was a feeding tube. "No!" we agreed in unison. There was no way we wanted to insert a tube down the nose all the way to the stomach. No, we were not going to do that no matter what. Our conversation went on and on. The last question was, in case you were about to die, would you prefer to die in the comfort of your home or at the hospital? "At the hospital," she said, adding that she didn't want us to live with the painful constant reminder if she was to leave us at home. Before we ended the conversation she asked if she could change her end-of-life care plans if her condition improved later on.

"Of course. You can change it anytime you want to," I quipped.

The following week was Samriddhi's regular post-chemo follow-up scan. She had been complaining of a dull ache in the nape of her neck. When she entered the blue doughnut tunnel, I stood at the corner, wearing a protective vest. Much to her annoyance, being away from her, even if it was for a short while was painful for us.

In between the whirring, buzzing, and clicking of the scan, I had a sinking feeling that the cancer had spread. The next morning, Ba (my father) and I went to collect the report.

I did not want to open the report. I did not want to know what was inside. But our house was only a two-minute walk away from the lab, and I needed to see the report and plan how to share it with Samriddhi. With the bold letters "METS" (Metastasis), the report showed that the tumor had spread further to the lungs and to the throat. When Ba kept asking me what the report said, I snapped that the report was not good. Right then, I decided to call the kennel club and get Samriddhi a pup. She had been wanting a dog for a long time.

"Who are you calling?" Ba asked in irritation.

"I'm getting a dog for Samriddhi," I yelled back.

"What are you talking about!" Ba exclaimed, trying to lower his voice.

"We're not all going to sit miserably because this report is ominous. We're going to decide how we feel every single second. We're getting a dog!!!" I screamed.

Often when we tried to set do's and don'ts for Samriddhi after she got cancer, she would get furious and tell us, including the doctors, that she was not going to let cancer define her life. That she would define her life on her own terms. Against medical advice while she was undergoing chemotherapy for brain cancer, Samriddhi flew to New Zealand. She wanted to see the first sunrise in the world and no one was going to stop her. It was the same with food. After our days-long stay at a cow therapy Ayurvedic center in Gujarat, they said she should only eat certain "alkaline" foods. But Samriddhi wanted to eat some chocolate cake and dare anyone stop her from doing just that. When life got out of control with cancer, Samriddhi took charge and controlled the things that she still could. Even if it was against medical advice or against our protective embrace, she did what felt right to her.

After back-to-back-to-back negative reports, I was done pegging my hopes on improving diagnostics. I was tired of Ma crying. I was tired of Ba howling. I was going to mirror Samriddhi—our lives would not be defined by cancer. Getting a pup seemed like a good place to start. When we got the baby dog home, Samriddhi named him Bhuntung. Not only because he was a round fluff ball but also because she wanted a name that she could pronounce clearly, even as her speech began to slur.

Gearing up for Travel

"And Daddy said, I am inside Taleju Bhawani temple. Tell Maami to come see me," my sister spoke in a groggy voice. Her eyes were still sleepy as she woke up from an afternoon nap.

Ma and I looked at one another, our eyes as big as headlights, taken aback at how Samriddhi had said that line in the exact same accent as Daddy. Daddy was our grandfather who we lost three years back. She even called our grandmother Maami, the name that only Daddy used. Both Samriddhi and I didn't know which temple Taleju Bhawani was until Ma explained that it was the one Daddy visited frequently, right in the heart of Kathmandu.

Samriddhi was now crying, pained by Daddy's memories and surprised to see him in her dream. Ma and I hugged her tight as she sat with her legs curled on the tilted hospital bed. Letting our guard down, we cried with her. I wasn't sure whether to be comforted that Daddy was looking out for her or if the dream meant she would be meeting Daddy soon. With the warm winter sun pouring in through the window, we hugged for a long time, sobbing silently, as the air tubes hissed inside the air mattress.

In her final months, Samriddhi regularly saw our late grandparents in her dreams. Sometimes our grandmother would visit and tell her that she would take all her pain away. Sometimes she said they were waiting for her and that she didn't have to worry at all. My father's parents had died long before Samriddhi and I were even born, so it always felt surreal that she would see them vividly in her dreams with such lucid messages.

That month when Samriddhi left us, the April of 2018, we frequently moved between the hospital and home. Ten days at the hospital, ten days at home, and then again ten days at the hospital. My sister never liked the hospital, so we would be keen on heading home hoping the change in environment would make her feel better. But with her condition deteriorating, we remained at the hospital. She slept most of the time and did not complain as much as she used to about going back home.

As we sat in the hospital room, a few weeks before we lost her, Samriddhi asked me to jot down a few things for her. I wasn't sure what she was asking me to note down, so I got a piece of paper and a pen. As she narrated, I listed down all the things she would need for her travel.

1. Face cream from The Body Shop
2. Two pairs of comfortable chappals—one with a horizontal flap and another the vertical kind
3. A small nail cutter
4. Earbuds
5. Wet wipes
6. Dove soap
7. Amla hair oil
8. Cotaryl cream for her hands
9. Zytee pain relief balm
10. A soft bristle toothbrush
11. Neem toothpaste
12. Mouthwash
13. Neosporin cream for the wounds inside her lips
14. A cream for rashes
15. Extra warm socks
16. Lip balm from The Body Shop
17. A large, soft towel and a small towel
18. Perfume

19. Wheelchair
20. Bedsheet
21. Blanket
22. Pillow

The list went on to include how we should clean and massage her face in case she could not do it on her own. I asked where she was traveling to, and she just replied that she would need all these things for her journey. From all the late night reading I did online when Samriddhi slept soundly, I knew that often before people die, they make a list of things to pack that they would need in their afterlife.

One afternoon, Samriddhi asked me for water but wasn't sure how to drink it when I gave her the small glass. By then, it seemed like her motor skills were somewhat affected. Confused, she dropped it. When she asked me for water again later, I held the glass for her, worried she would drop it again. But she was reluctant. She wanted to drink on her own. Almost knowing what was on my mind, she asked me to move back, behind her. I gave her a look that said, "No, Samriddhi," but she insisted. I caved in and did as she wanted me to, taking a few steps back. Samriddhi waited until she felt I was a safe distance away and smash, threw the glass on the floor. I started laughing. Why would she throw the glass? Despite everything going on inside her, she was so thoughtful that she made sure I was at a safe distance before throwing the glass. Samriddhi laughed after me, imitating my reaction as if she was a little baby imitating the adults around her. I kissed her hands.

In the final week all we did was kiss Samriddhi and tell her we loved her. I would ask her, "Do you love Baba?" Unable to open her mouth and speak, Samriddhi would nod her head like a little baby looking at my father. When I asked, "Can he kiss your hand?" she would nod again. And we would kiss her hands a million times, massage her legs, and her hands as we had always done, even when they stopped moving on their own.

For as Long as We Live, You Will Be Loved

"Can you please take Bhuntung to your room? The electrician is here to fix the oven," Ba asked as I was concentrating hard on slicing the cucumbers into thin perfect circles.

"Hyaa... just ask Samriddhi!" I snapped, looking up from my chopping board.

We stared at each other in utter shock. Silence. It had been four years since we had lost my sister. A few seconds later, when my mind was able to make sense of what had just come out of my mouth. "Just ask Ma," I managed to mumble and dashed out of the kitchen, squeezing Bhuntung tight in my arms.

A million daggers come out of nowhere, stabbing me with reality, painfully reminding me of how life could have been had Samriddhi still been around. Out of the long list of things that I could think of, clearly, the first was dividing our chores equally!

I still remember that in the early days after we lost Samriddhi, one of the most difficult things to do was to sit at the dining table and eat. To put food inside your mouth while Samriddhi's seat was empty was torturous. I'm not sure how each of us processed the pain. Ma would be the first to start crying, followed by Ba. We would just sit and cry, biting on our rotis between sobs and painful gulps.

We kept a beautiful sketch of Samriddhi right in the center of our living room. It's like an altar where we keep flowers, candles, a glass of water, and small plates of food for every meal. For Ma, the sketch came to represent Samriddhi. She would fall asleep on the sofa every night staring at it. I would come from my room, coax her, scold her, and sometimes even pull her to go to bed and sleep inside her room. Sometimes I managed to do so by 10 p.m., but on other occasions she would refuse to budge and kept trying till 1 am. With passing years, this ritual of waking Ma up and insisting she sleep inside her room has become less frequent.

While with Ma, I would be doubly patient, I couldn't keep up when it came to Ba. Handling my own emotions and those of Ma was already a lot for me to manage. I would unfairly snap when Ba lost his composure. Whenever Ma was not home, he would look at Samriddhi's videos and secretly pine. I counted on Avi, my close friends, and cousins to support Ba as I felt I did not have the energy to support one more parent. All of us had to focus on looking after Ma as she was the only one who did not have an alternate identity after Samriddhi left us. The rest of us, Ba, Avi, and I had full-time jobs to return to. Jobs that we were passionate about, jobs that forced us out of our homes every day and got us involved in luxuries such as mundane everyday activities and little workplace dramas. But Ma had retired from her job when Samriddhi's cancer had returned, and her only identity was that of Samriddhi's primary caretaker.

Life had come to a sudden standstill for all of us. We were doing everything we could, and some more, to look after Samriddhi when she was with us. Even after we lost her, we followed many rituals in the hope that it would make a difference. But we were desperate, to do everything in our power, to continue loving and caring for her, just the way we did when she was with us. As a means to help us keep her spirit alive, we decided to fulfill one of Samriddhi's wishes of giving back to Sisaut—my father's ancestral home. Samriddhi had always wanted to visit, but we always had to keep putting it off for later, for when she would recover. We decided to establish a foundation in Sisaut in her memory. We called it the Puku Didi Foundation. Puku is a nickname my parents had fondly given to Samriddhi. On what would've been Samriddhi's 30th birthday, we started the foundation by supporting two girls in Sisaut with scholarships. Today, under Ma's leadership, the foundation supports more than 15 girls in Sisaut to go to school and is taking on bigger initiatives.

Many times, confused students ask us, "Ma'am... Who exactly is Puku Didi?" tearing us up. We are always overcome with emotions when someone decides to support the foundation, moved by their love for Samriddhi. It is an incredible feeling that Samriddhi lives on through the foundation, spreading her love and light and influencing lives for the better beyond our family and Sisaut across Nepal.

—Subeksha Poudel

WHEN A CAREGIVER GETS CANCER

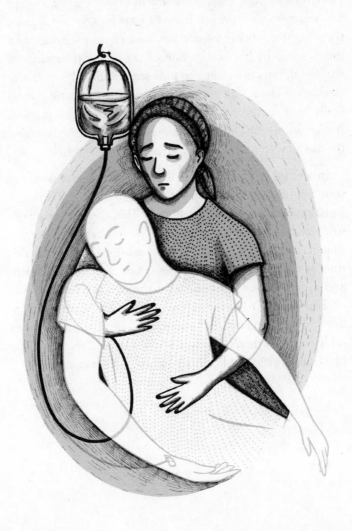

It's extremely challenging to be a caregiver to a patient. At the end of a tumultuous journey, there are only two outcomes, you either see your loved one come out free of this disease or you see them pass away in front of your eyes. In some cases, they might get better briefly but have to keep getting treatment regularly. It's like a game of tag. Their treatments, if successful, buys them time to hide for a while, till the cancer catches up again. This cycle continues for a while, till it eventually captures them for good. That is the end of their game. It takes a long time but you finally grow around your grief and the loss of your loved one becomes a part of your life.

In a weird twist of fate, life then throws another googly at you. You get diagnosed yourself and are left asking if losing a loved one to cancer wasn't enough. This is every caregiver's worst nightmare come true, apart from another loved one getting diagnosed. You go through the motions again, only this time as a patient yourself. You now understand all the pain and suffering your loved one went through and was trying to explain to you. You worry about ending up the same way as them, dying prematurely. You secretly keep hoping that your odds are better than theirs were. Take a look at what life looks like from the other side, once you have been a caregiver.

CHANGING TIDES

Donning my graduation gown and headdress, I gazed across and caught the look on Mum's face—a mix of adulation, pride, and happy tears. My graduation truly meant the world to her—she had supported my desire to pursue hospitality management and I had done it! She cheered loudly and proudly when my name was announced. I was feeling euphoric yet emotional to see her this joyful, knowing that deep down inside she was battling with the scars of being a breast cancer patient. But never did she let it show when she had to be there for her children. It was a milestone moment for her to witness her eldest child graduating, far away from our hometown Singapore, in picturesque Switzerland. She could temporarily escape the stresses of life back home and have a "mother-daughter holiday." These were some of our most cherished moments together.

Sigh. If only they could last forever. Having settled back in Singapore after the graduation holiday, inevitably I had to accompany her for a routine scan. She expressed a lot of anxiety about the scan once we returned. I quickly realized that the emotional "highs" of the vacation had worn off and there was a mental burden she struggled to shake off. Being young, I trivialized her worries by simply assuring her that everything would be fine.

However, life had other plans for us. The scan results had anomalies that required further investigation and this left Mum in a state of uncertainty. Further tests concluded that the cancer had metastasized to her liver and further surgery and chemotherapy were the necessary next step. My heart sank. My family was devastated. I was very attached to Mum and could not bear that she had to face the whole ordeal again. She had just escaped this reality while we were in Switzerland and it had barely taken a few days back home for it all to come crashing down, with a dark tunnel of unknown lying ahead of us. This time—from the look in her eyes—I could sense that she was overwhelmed, anxious, and miserable. She needed me now more than ever before to be by her side. Willingly, instead of starting a career, I prioritized supporting her in every way I could. The role of being a caregiver for her was far more meaningful than any job. My two younger siblings were still in school, so I needed to ease some of my father's burden.

From thereon began my journey as a caregiver—to witness the toll of cancer on a person you love. The never-ending visits to medical care facilities and managing the side effects of chemotherapy. The brutally honest feedback from doctors who were trying their best but never quite feeling fully assured that their best would be enough.

Despite our efforts, the disease was not deterred and my mother's condition began to deteriorate. My family retained the hope that she would find a way or that the treatment would eventually work in our favor. But it didn't. I remember that fateful night at home when she could no longer continue to fight. We gathered around her and whispered our goodbyes in her final moments. I held her hand as she faded away.

Holding my mother while she withered away was one of the most painful and heartbreaking things I had ever experienced. While I felt a certain degree of relief that she was no longer suffering, I struggled to find solace. I missed her all the time. I missed the way she smiled, the way her fingers felt were when she held my hand, the unconditional love I experienced when she used to stroke my head and hug me. It was a love that could only come from a mother.

My family felt disoriented for months after. Grief hit us every now and then in the most unexpected of times. My father had to take on the role of being both a father and a mother to us three children. It took us all a long time to heal. All of us were a little lost in our own ways, yet we needed to find our own recourse to move forward.

Six months later, an angel entered my life when I least expected it. I met a guy at a friend's wedding. He reached out after the wedding and I was open to the idea of getting to know him better. How kind he was, always listening to me and always being there for me, uplifting my spirits and bringing back my smile with his witty humor. I started feeling cheerful and happy again, something I had not felt in a long time. One year later, he proposed. Wow! What a beautiful proposal, on a boat (from where, he said, I would have nowhere to run! haha!), in the middle of the Singapore river.

After a long period of depression and grief, things were finally looking up! I remember how much Mum wanted me to settle down and marry a man from a good family and with a kind heart. I looked up at the stars and saw one shining brighter than the rest that night—I took comfort in knowing that maybe it was a sign of Mum giving her blessing. It meant a lot to me. I often looked out for signs of her in moments that involved a decision or an action or even while being in a place that I knew she would have enjoyed being in. It was my way of coping with her absence, my way of feeling that she is watching over me—just like that gaze I caught on my graduation day.

I was thrilled to plan my wedding. I had so many ideas about everything, from what I would wear to how we would plan the festivities and with whom we would celebrate. What could possibly go wrong now? Or so I thought.

It had been almost two years since Mum's passing. Both my sister and I were aware that we ought to check our breasts for anything unusual. Subconsciously, I would just do it every few months. Little did I know that a simple action like that could save my life. One night, during a routine self-check, I felt a lump on my right breast.

"What, where did that come from?" I had not felt it before. I'd imagine most young women would typically ignore it but with my experience, I consulted a doctor immediately and was advised to get additional tests done.

"But it cannot be, I am so young" I brushed it off reassuring myself it was probably a cyst. A week later the biopsy confirmed my worst fears—Stage 2A breast cancer. How could that be possible! We just lost Mum to cancer two years ago and now I had it? Please God help me. Feelings of dread, anger, betrayal, and sadness took over. I was only 25 years old and always been relatively healthy. What could have caused it? Was it the emotional grief and stress from losing Mum? Was it my diet? Or karma of my past birth? So many unanswered questions clouded my mind.

We decided to consult the same doctor who had been treating Mum. I felt such an eerie sense of déjà vu as I sat in the same chair that my mother used to sit on. From being a caregiver and accompanying Mum for her treatments, I had now become the recipient of the treatment with my family, and my fiancé had been forced to take on the caregiver's role. I felt the universe was playing a cruel joke on us. I was terrified because I had already been a first-hand witness to how cancer could withstand the toughest treatment regimens planned by the best doctors in the world. My mind constantly wondered if I was meant to tread the same path my mother had trodden.

But it wasn't just about me either. How was I to tell my fiancé that I had breast cancer? Would this be the very first hurdle we had to go through together? Or would he not want to marry me? What would happen to my hair after the chemotherapy and what about our wedding plans? –With tears trickling down, I had a vulnerable conversation with my fiancé, less than three months after his proposal. He reassured me, "We are in this together. We will face whatever comes our way." I admired his emotional maturity for making the decision to stand by me, knowing that this would affect our marriage, the prospect of ever having children, and even my identity. There were times I sensed my fiancé was holding back tears, but he was a man loyal to his promise to stand by me as he had vowed in his proposal—"In this life, you will face more battles than what you were supposed to, but from now on we'll make them ours and overcome them together."

Indeed, our love would have to stand the harshest of trials. Cycle after cycle of chemotherapy, side effect after side effect. What was meant to be the engagement period filled with celebratory meets with our relatives and friends was soon filled with never-ending doctor appointments and weekly hospital visits.

I saw flashbacks of Mum. I remembered how she had decided to shave off the hair on her head before starting chemotherapy. Back then, I disagreed with her and couldn't understand her decision but here I was now in that very position. A few weeks into chemo, I tried not to comb my hair, thinking it would not drop. Instead, my hair began to stiffen and would fall out in clumps. I stared at the mirror and knew that I had to make the same decision she had made. That night, I asked my father to cut my hair short.

My wedding had to be postponed by a year. I needed the time after treatment to regain my energy. Up to this point, I had kept my condition very private and stayed out of the public eye. My family was not comfortable that I reveal the challenges I was going through to anyone outside of a close-knit circle. So that is what I did. Even when I lost my hair, I didn't speak about it to anyone beyond my family and very close friends. It was suffocating. I was in denial for a very long time. Moreover, I was raised to believe that it was not "right" to seek professional therapy so I dealt with my mental state on my own. However, the truth is this trauma was unique and I didn't know how to help myself.

After six months of harsh chemotherapy, a mastectomy, and reconstruction of the right breast, eventually a PET scan showed no cancer in the body. In other words, I was in REMISSION! That was a magic word. To be in remission after the grueling months meant that I could finally end chemotherapy and could move forward in my life. What a magnificent feeling. My fiancé and I kickstarted the wedding preparations from where we had left off. I felt good again. I felt like we were returning to somewhat scarred but mostly normal lives where we can focus on ourselves and be happy again.

Our wedding happened on the most gorgeous day—clear blue skies and a joyous atmosphere surrounded us. Our friends and family were in full attendance, giving us their blessings and applauding this milestone. As I stood next to the man who endured it all by my side—truly giving meaning to the vows in sickness and health forsaking all others—I felt it was one of the happiest days of my life. Together we celebrated our wedding, and in our hearts, we celebrated the fact that I had beaten cancer.

Married life began. We kept to our routines and monitored our health through exercise, conscious dieting, and medical follow-ups. However, at the back of my mind a nagging feeling of worry remained that I could never fully shake off. Could I actually have been cured? I would easily get triggered by any subsequent symptom or unusual ache which would send me in a state of panic and prompt me to ask, "Is the cancer back?" I wanted to believe that I had defeated it, but I somehow never fully could.

The years were going by quickly. I had been taking hormonal pills daily for four and a half years. I was so close to the milestone five-year mark that every cancer survivor waits for. I felt good as my scans had been clear so far. For me, reaching the five-year mark meant a reassurance that the chances of recurrence had become much lower. More importantly, it would mean my husband and I could finally begin to plan our family. We decided that we would first wait for the results of my upcoming scan. However, I was already dreaming. I had already picked out names for a baby boy and a baby girl. I had already mentally started visualizing how I wanted to design the nursery in our home. I spoke to my father about how he would spend his time with a grandchild as ours would be the first for him. How exciting it was!

The twists and turns that cancer had in store for us were not over, though. The follow-up scan brought up a nodule in the lung which eventually after a biopsy confirmed my worst fear—the cancer had metastasized. Now, I was a Stage 4 metastatic breast cancer patient. Everything changed immediately. I went through the roller coaster of emotions once again, depression and anger being at the forefront.

"Why again? Why me God? What did I do to deserve this? Am I not meant to be happy?"

From the moment I heard Stage 4, it was all I could think of. My worst nightmare had come true. It haunted me every waking moment, "Stage 4, Stage 4, Stage 4". Flashes of Mum kept coming into my thoughts. "Am I going to face the same fate that she did?" It felt as if I was racing against time. How did my life turn out this way at 30? I could not help but compare myself with my peers who were moving forward in their lives, while I had to start chemotherapy again and face a life of seemingly endless uncertainties.

Those were some of the darkest days of my life. I felt so alone. Even with my family there to support me, I felt nobody could fully comprehend my feelings. I felt extremely guilty that my family had to go through this again and felt like a burden to everyone around me. In the blink of an eye, instead of moving forward, I was moving backward. Being Stage 4 meant I would be on some form of treatment indefinitely.

The treatment plan was set—four cycles of chemotherapy followed by a scan. We would reevaluate to see if we would continue the same regimen or change it. It was a game of trial and error which would determine the future of my life.

What hurt me the most was that I was advised against having children as my cancer was fueled by hormones and a pregnancy would be counterproductive to the hormonal management needs that my treatment required. I felt devastated that I was so close to the five-year mark of remission and yet so far away. I was angry at the universe, at my body, and even at God.

Treatment for relapse was challenging. The chemotherapy lasted for nine months. Cycle after cycle, I experienced immense side effects with body aches. I often faced the loaded question, "Is this all worth it?" And the answer has been the same, "Yes, it is."

Post chemotherapy, I thought life would go back to normal but my body was dealing with the cumulative effect of treatment and needed lots of rest, tender love, and care. It took me one full year before I felt remotely close to normal.

Currently, to keep my health stable I have to undergo maintenance treatment which means an antibodies injection has to be taken every three weeks. At times, I still struggle to accept this reality. I still deal with the many side effects that come along with my treatment and it is difficult as I can never predict how I am going to feel. Every day brings some new challenges that I have to physically deal with.

I make peace with the fact that I came into this life for a purpose, one that was bigger than what I thought it would be and as much as I can, I am here to share my story. Despite all that has happened, I do my best to live in the present moment and enjoy the day in front of me. I do things that keep me happy. I travel, eat, and try not to worry about things that don't serve me. I don't ponder as much about the future and what might happen but rather make memories with the people I love. In some ways, I have accepted the fact that my mother and I are two different souls and our fates don't necessarily have to be the same.

I hold on to hope that in the near future someone will find a silver bullet to cure cancer and that a miracle is waiting just around the corner. I would like to think that I am a survivor so far and that there is always a reason why things happen the way they do, even if I don't fully understand it. I will make the most of what life allows me to.

—Nikita Wadhwani

THE REAL AND
THE SURREAL

I still remember the day we brought my grandfather home from
the hospital. He had just undergone surgery to remove a tumor
from his spine. We got him out of the ambulance and put him in
his bed. And then there was a flood.

No, I don't mean a flood of emotions.

An actual flood, with water rushing in through the gate and
under the door. As my grandfather lay in bed, I watched the water
slowly filling his room. If you were to make a list of all the emotions one is likely to feel in a moment like this, mild amusement
would probably not be on it. Yet there I was, mildly amused at the
predicament my family was in. As if watching a man in his nineties
going through a major surgery wasn't enough, we now had to deal
with a flooding house. It almost seemed like we were in a movie
where the characters had to go through surreal experiences to pass
some character test. You know, your average feel-good god works in
mysterious ways fable.

Like all stories, this story too must begin somewhere. Let us
begin at the very beginning, when I had my first brush with cancer. Cancer, the emperor of all maladies, is something we hope we
never have to encounter personally. For me at least, it was always
something that affected other people. I knew of relatives who had

it and celebrities who got treated for it but I always maintained an emotional distance from it. That was until my grandfather was diagnosed. It was in 2008 that my then eighty-two-year-old grandfather was diagnosed with throat cancer, which always brings to mind the anti-tobacco ads we are made to watch before the movies start. Someone had to sell their gold bangles because they ate gutkha (chewing tobacco). It came as a surprise that my grandfather who had never smoked or chewed gutkha had throat cancer. The cancer had come home and it didn't even ring the bell. Well, at least no one heard it at first.

My grandfather, a retired police officer who had no major ailments to speak of and was one of the fittest eighty-two-year-olds I have ever seen, gradually began to lose his voice. We lived away from home at that time but could notice his voice changing over the phone. As his voice kept getting worse, all roads led us towards the Mordor of hospitals, the oncology department. Oncology departments are surreal places because of their liminality. Many people who step into them fear the worst. Patients there are just one scan away from living a normal life or being yanked into cancer treatment. Here's what it's like to be in there—one of the leading cancer hospitals in the country has installed nets, and no, they are not for volleyball. Of course, you could also argue that people there are just one scan away from being declared cancer-free but my point is that oncology wards have always felt surreal to me. I had always hoped that I would never have to go to one but you know what they say, wish upon a star and you'll get a tumor.

Speaking of tumors, here's a nice transition to my grandfather's diagnosis. Once we found out that he had cancer, we had no choice but to get the surgery done immediately. That's the thing about cancer, everything is okay until suddenly it's not. So, there we were thinking about subjecting my grandfather to a major surgery. Mind you, everything becomes a major surgery when you're in your eighties. But as the saying goes, you have to risk it to get the biscuit and so risk it we did. Don't get me wrong, we didn't just blindly go with the first surgeon we found. After seeking many opinions, we closed in on the best man for the job, an ear, nose, and throat surgeon who was the best in the game. As far as surgeries go, this one was something out of a Tarantino movie. So, here's the deal with tumors. You can't really diagnose whether they are dangerous or not until you have a piece of the actual tumor. Generally, a biopsy is performed on a sample before deciding on the next course of treatment. In my grandfather's case, we had to make this decision while he was on the operating table.

Due to his advanced age, it was too risky to put him under anesthesia twice, so it was decided that the biopsy would be done while he was on the table, and based on the results, they would decide what to do next. Time for a plot twist. The biopsy could only be done at a specific lab, which was in another part of the city. Enter the hero, my dad. It was decided that he would personally deliver the sample to the lab using the fastest possible mode of transport—a Scooty. So, I guess TVS is the real hero here. On the day of the surgery, the doctors and my dad orchestrated one of the best-planned tumor heists in the world. My dad planned out the job to the minute and executed it perfectly, but the results of the biopsy were anything but.

It was decided that my grandfather would have to lose his voice box. He went into the theatre after eighty-two years of using a voice box and came out without one. His voice box was replaced with a tracheostomy speaking valve. Simply put, a hole in his neck. He would have to train himself to speak again. I remember how surreal it was visiting him in the ICU and seeing him communicating with a slate. But before we get to the good part, we must endure the horrifying parts, like the night we almost lost him. The details are hazy, but soon after the surgery, the hole on my grandfather's neck started spewing blood. I don't mean bleeding, I mean spewing. Because it was in the early hours of the morning, the surgeon was able to rush across Bengaluru in eight minutes. The stuff of action movies. We would have probably lost my grandfather if it weren't for him. My dad, who saw it happen, must have said his goodbyes.

My grandfather, being the badass he was, was able to recover his voice without ever making us feel that it was a difficult transition for him. He lived for another ten years. Divine intervention.

The second time around, it finally got him. My grandfather had always been a fighter, but the second time I could see him losing the fight and the sudden deterioration was stunning. One day he was going about his daily routine, in great shape considering he was ninety-two, and the next we were calling an ambulance. This time the tumor came back with friends and the worst of them were in his spine. I will never forget the night we took him to the hospital. He had lost control of his bladder and lay there in his urine. The hospital didn't even have the decency to change his bedding. I can't even begin to imagine how he must have felt. This is a man who meticulously groomed himself and wore crisp shirts he ironed himself even in his nineties. Oh, and the doctor didn't tell us that unless he underwent surgery, my grandfather could lose control of his bladder and perhaps his mobility for life. Oops, I guess he forgot. Shit happens. Needless to say, we didn't feel safe at that hospital and decided to shift him.

So, it was under these circumstances that my grandfather went under the scalpel for a second time. In a perfect world, no one would subject a ninety-two-year-old to spinal surgery, but we didn't have a choice. At least the choices we had were like Sophie's choices. If we didn't choose surgery, he was looking at living the rest of his life without mobility and control of his bladder. Surgery offered some hope that he would have a better quality of life. What would you choose?

When he went into the operation theatre that day, I wasn't sure I'd see him again. But he made it out at least. The mobility that the surgery was supposed to preserve never came back. In fact, the day that we took him to the hospital was the last time he walked. The next few months are a blur because every day was the same. Mark, the nurse we hired, and I trying to get my grandfather to regain some semblance of his old life back. We would carry him out to the garden, pick him up, and get him to walk. we repeated this every day, until the days leading up to his passing. On some nights I would sit by his bedside and weep. This was my first encounter with someone dying. The whole process is so otherworldly. You keep hoping that there will be a recovery but one day you start to realize that this might be it. On his last day, I stepped out for a haircut. In the middle of it, I got a call that he was leaving. I rushed home and gave him a sip of water. He held on to life till I came back as if he was waiting for me to say goodbye. Then, he passed away. I would like to say that we had time to process the grief, but as soon as he passed away, we had to attend to many bureaucratic and ritualistic things—arrange a death certificate, arrange a priest, arrange the cremation, etc., you know the drill. Well actually, I hope you don't. A loud pop from the funeral pyre signaled that my grandfather's soul had left his body and that was that. That was my second encounter with cancer.

Cancer came back into my life for a third time, this time in my own body. It sounds silly, but I honestly never believed that I would get it. I'm not too morbid or anything, just as morbid as your average next-door guy, but I had thought about what I would do if I ever got it. In my head, it was a bucket list kind of situation, where I would cycle around the world, jump off a plane, and leave the world with my middle finger pointing to the sky. But turns out, so far, it's mostly been sliding into MRI machines and out of hospitals. One of the worst things about cancer (other than cancer itself) in my experience is how suddenly your life changes. One day you're going about your life and the next day you're a cancer patient.

My journey began with a cycle ride. Before you send out a WhatsApp forward, no cycling does not cause cancer, just piles. I got into cycling during the COVID-19 pandemic and it has now really become one of my favorite things so much so that it is now a personality trait. If we ever meet, I'll probably tell you I'm a cyclist before we get to the third sentence. Anyway, during one of my morning rides, I stopped for a coffee and I collapsed. Twice in under a minute. My friend brought me home, and we rushed to my eye doctor. What does an eye doctor have to do with passing out would be a natural question to ask. That's a story for another book, but the short answer is that an ophthalmologist was treating me for idiopathic intracranial hypertension (IIH) for a while. If you want to learn more about that, you'll have to buy my next book. When I collapsed a week after completing my treatment, our first thought was that maybe the IIH was acting up. But we were wrong. Turns out I had a tumor in my neck that was blocking blood flow. To figure out what type of tumor it was, we had to ask the saddest sounding board of all time, the tumor board.

Though the brains of the tumor board concluded that what I had might be benign, we decided that I would undergo a biopsy because I got tired of playing, will it kill me, will it kill me not? The worst part was that my tumor was in a really difficult-to-access place. For the biopsy, a neuroradiologist would have to insert a needle into my neck and extract a sample. Cue Mission Impossible music. Needle in, sample out. Pretty simple, right? Except for one small detail. In case the needle hit a nerve or something, there could be some pretty serious consequences. I had to lay completely still while the procedure was performed and to my credit, I managed fine. To the doctor's credit, he executed it perfectly. Now that we had a sample, we could finally find out what I actually had. And boy, did we get some bad news. I had something called a chondroid chordoma, a slow-growing, rare, and dangerous tumor. In the interests of honesty, I hadn't panicked until then. But it was time to change that. My mind went to some pretty dark places and I'd rather not shed light on those places here. Suffice to say, the trauma box is overflowing at this point.

Once the boat crossed the acceptance bridge, it took a sharp right turn towards the action jetty. Surgical removal is the best possible solution, so now it was my time to shine. How does one choose a surgeon for something like this? Google reviews would be a good starting place. Anything below 4.6 is best avoided. Till this point, I had some agency but someone else was the captain now. All I could do was live my life and prepare for D-Day. In the days leading up to the surgery, I did everything as if I wasn't sure I'd be able to do it again. Was I being a little dramatic? Maybe, but do I feel bad about it? Hell no. Okay, we can skip the ad now.

I woke up in the ICU without any tubes sticking out of my throat. Take that consent form that warns of "theoretical risks to life." But my celebrations were short-lived. If you have ever wondered about the human propensity to vomit, wonder no more. The answer is very high. The post-op days were spent holding on to my bed for dear life because I would vomit if I sat up. Standing was a stretch and walking would have meant asking a fish to climb a tree. Mornings were the worst because I had to bathe while on pretty strong drugs. And they weren't even the fun kind. I somehow managed to find the strength to leave the hospital after seven days of recreating all the best of Jackson Pollock's works with my bodily fluids. I lay down on the backseat of the car and looked at the city passing by and thought to myself "damn that was pretty wild."

As I write this, I am preparing for the next step of my treatment. I will have to undergo something called cyberknife therapy. Some Russian hackers will stab my brain or something like that. The surgeons did a pretty good job and removed most of the tumor and the cyberknife will remove the rest of it. As I'm looking for a way to end this chapter, the universe answers. I can see the water rushing into my house from underneath the door. It's flooding again. I couldn't make this shit up if I tried.

—Aditya Arun

ACKNOWLEDGEMENTS

Firstly, I'd like to express my heartfelt gratitude to the commissioning editor of our book, my dear friend Chandrima Chatterjee, for her generous support. No matter what time or day of the week it was, she has been there throughout the process of envisioning, organizing, writing, editing, and producing this book. Without her, this would have been just another crazy idea, an unticked item on my bucket list, and an unfulfilled dream. So, thank you Chandrima for helping me wet my feet in the world of authoring books. I hope this will finally give me the courage to write and publish more, including the memoir that I have been dreaming of writing.

Secondly, I want to sincerely acknowledge Saumita Banerjee and her open authoring platform LetsAuthor, which gave me the opportunity to work on and publish this very urgent and necessary book. I wonder if any mainstream publication would have bet their money on someone who has never published anything before and a book with such a select audience. So, thank you for putting your faith in me and for all the support you and your team have provided.

I'd also like to express my deepest appreciation for all the co-authors from across the country and the world who believed in my vision and trusted me to get this book organized, written, and published. I cannot thank all of you enough for being so vulnerable in your writing, taking my feedback constructively, and revising your drafts multiple times in the hope that the final chapters will help thousands of others who may find themselves in your shoes.

I'd like to let all our backers know how indebted we are to their support. By funding the publication of this book you've done a great service in helping these stories reach the underserved young adult cancer community. This book will help our community feel acknowledged and represented in the sea of cancer self-help books that don't actually address any of our issues or help us in any concrete way at all. Your endorsement will also help those whose experiences and narratives have often been ignored and marginalized, consciously and unconsciously, by many of us.

A quick note of thanks to our brilliant illustrator and my dear friend Suman Kaur who agreed to help me out with beautiful theme-based illustrations and author portraits in a short period of time, without getting frustrated with my nagging to meet our deadlines. I'd also like to thank Manoj Vijayan for designing our gorgeous book cover. Thank you both for elevating our stories with your stunning visuals.

Finally, I am grateful to all those who will buy this book for themselves or someone they know who has been touched by cancer, I hope that it's just a brush with and not a kiss of death. We collectively wish no one experiences this ailment, not even our nemeses. In case you'd like to contact us for anything, including finding support or sharing feedback on the book, please feel free to reach out to us at dontaskmebook@gmail.com. We'll try to respond at the earliest.

—Sanjay Deshpande

ABOUT THE AUTHORS

Sanjay Deshpande (Lead Author)

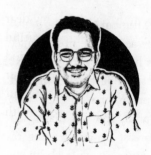

Sanjay is a brain cancer survivor who was diagnosed at the age of 29 on the day he landed on Harvard University's campus to start his master's in September 2021.

He is a learning designer who is passionate about mental health and queer rights. He loves to dance and try different cuisines. He hopes to write a memoir and travel the world before he kicks the bucket.

He's leading the effort to publish this book to raise awareness about the unique challenges faced by Indian young adult cancer patients, survivors and caregivers. He currently lives in Hyderabad with his parents.

Sachin Rajakrishnan

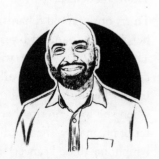

Sachin is an aviation geek who loves working in the aviation industry. His recently acquired label of cancer survivor has allowed him to reflect on the shortness and the beauty of life in a more personal manner, and he is determined to savor the colors of life that cancer revealed to him every single day.

He is passionate about nature and wildlife conservation and hopes to be able to fully contribute to them someday. He also loves reading fantasy books and playing board games and hopes to author an epic fantasy and create a spectacular board game.

He is also the sidekick to his wonder woman wife, Divya; chief storyteller and dad-Vader to his two Jedi sons, Shiv and Shyam; and canine of equal rank to his beautiful Labrador, Iris.

Snehal Ponde

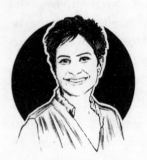

Growing up in Mumbai and living a hectic corporate life as an HR professional, Snehal and her husband had their next adventure charted out as they moved to Singapore, pregnant with their first child. Shortly after, she was diagnosed with Stage 4 breast cancer, leading to a rollercoaster journey, while she navigated her treatment as a new mother, in a new country. As the wait to be cancer-free kept extending, with the support of her loved ones, she slowly pieced her life together. She is now a coach and motivational speaker, empowering others to take charge and own their story.

Thanisha Sehgal

Thirty-one-year-old Thanisha stays with her husband and two-year-old son in Thailand. At 29, she was living her dream life, excelling at work, and preparing for her upcoming motherhood. Just when she was entering her third trimester of pregnancy, she was diagnosed with lymphoma (blood cancer). Life has never been the same since.

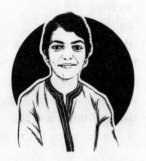

Two years after the diagnosis and multiple rounds of chemo and radiation, today she is cancer free. She is a product management professional who, during leisure hours, likes to bake, listen to and sing along nursery rhymes, and is deeply interested in parenthood. She wants to tell her story of struggles, failures, victories and stories of thriving to many like her, in the hope that she can make them feel warm and belonged.

Anuraag Khaund

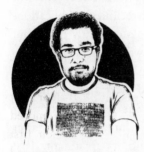

Anuraag Khaund is a Homo Sapiens from Guwahati, Assam, with an avid interest in history, culture, and international relations. He was diagnosed with Chronic Myeloid Leukemia (CML) in 2021, an experience that gave him a new perspective on life, health, family, and religion. Hence, he answered the call by LetsAuthor to share his newfound experiences and epiphany with muggles and other cancer newbies. Besides his temper, another major drawback of Anuraag is his habit of turning every form of writing into boring academic lectures. However, he believes the chapters in this book bring out his fun side along with the serious, boring one.

Piuli Roy Choudhury

Piuli is a finance professional who recently migrated to Frankfurt. She enjoys long walks, dark humor, travels that surprise and shock, and reading fiction. Although professionally trained in Bharatnatyam for over fifteen years, she now prefers the informality of dancing at friends' weddings.

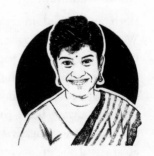

She spent three months as a caregiver to her brother who was diagnosed with a type of blood cancer called T-ALL (T-cell Acute Lymphoblastic Leukemia) in April 2021. She chose to contribute to this book in the hope of finding closure as well as sharing her story with other caregivers who may find themselves in the same boat.

Vani Verma

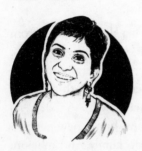

Vani Verma is a breast cancer survivor who works as a technical publications professional. She is currently based out of Toronto. She was diagnosed with the disease at the age of 31, right before she had to land and start her journey in a new country. She learned about her BRCA 1 genetic mutation only after getting cancer and its treatment. Post numerous surgeries including a prophylactic bilateral mastectomy, she continues to sing and chat wholeheartedly.

She loves to bask in the sun and cook meals. You will occasionally find her without a smile on her face and a sensitive thought in her head.

Nikita Wadhwani

Born and raised in Singapore, Nikita Wadhwani was diagnosed with early breast cancer at the young age of 25, three months after being engaged to her fiancé. She loves the simple things in life and has always been passionate about reading and writing. Travel is her way to escape and she enjoys rediscovering and finding parts of herself. She had a relapse and is now currently living

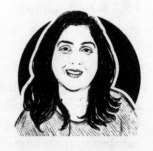

as a metastatic breast cancer survivor and wants to share her story with young survivors who are going through similar experiences.

Pallavi Saraswatula

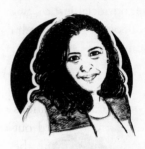

Pallavi would describe herself as a jack of all trades. A qualified lawyer, she was diagnosed with cancer before she could truly establish herself professionally. While it was unfortunate, she didn't want to constantly think of herself as a cancer survivor. So, during her treatments, she used the time on her hands to learn new hobbies she'd always wanted to try, and now she has knowledge in fields ranging from graphic designing, animation, editing, upcycling, crocheting, and resin art. Writing about her journey was always been something she'd wanted to do, and with this book, she finally got the chance.

Aditya Arun

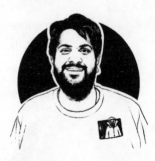

Aditya practices instructional design and it pays for his other passions. One day he hopes to pursue his passions full time, becoming a travel writer, baker-barista cyclist. Though he has always been a storyteller at heart, writing became his North Star during the dark days when he was diagnosed with a rare malignant tumor called a Chondroid Chordoma. He hopes his writing will bring a smile to someone's face, once they stop judging him for writing about himself in the third person. At the time of writing this book, he was undergoing treatment for his tumor and will soon be able to celebrate being cancer free.

Subeksha Poudel

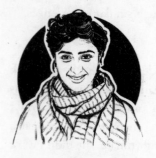

Subeksha is a passionate feminist and a communications professional. Through her work, she advocates for intersectional feminism and social justice. She holds a Master of Sociology from Delhi School of Economics.

Poornima Sardana

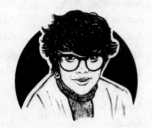

Poornima Sardana is a curator and museum consultant based in New Delhi. She is interested in the intersection of care, health, and culture. A Fulbright-Nehru alumna, she researches and experiments with museums' contribution to society's well-being, particularly emotional, through her initiative Museums of Hope.

LIST OF BACKERS

Aadi Vaidya
Aaditya Rawat
Aakanksha Pandey
Aakankshi Javeri
Aakankshya Das
Aakash Batra
Aanchal Sacheti
Aaradhyaa Kaviyarasu
Aarti Bisla
Aarti Samay Mantri
Aashish DMello
Aashna Gutgutia
Abdul Riaz Nazeer
Abhas Kumat
Abhijit Kachhap
Abhinandan Saikia
Abhinay Bhasin
Abhisha Shrivastava
Abhishek Bansal
Abhishek Ghosh
Abhishek Mishra
Abhishek Sarda
Achintya Prahlad
Adith Anande
Aditi Kulkarni
Aditi Maiti
Aditya Arun

Aditya Raja
Aditya Chakravarty
Aditya Samtani
Agrima Nagpal
Aheed Khan
Aishwarya Parammal Upot
Ajay Herur
Ajay Kalra
Ajay Rudraraju
Akanksha Trivedi
Akhilesh Kumar Verma
Akshay Lakhi
Akshi Gundamraj
Ali Baig
Alishuba Philip
Alok Panigrahy
Alok Patel
Aman Arora
Aman Dubey
Amarendra Katkar
Ameya Kulkarni
Amol Khedkar
Amrish Sawe
Amrita Khemlani
Anagha Ganti
Anam Zaidi
Anand Jeyasekharan

Anand Kannan
Ananya Bhatia
Ananya Singh
Anderson Glashan
Andrea Nevay
Anindya Basu
Anjali Shekhar
Anjana Rajendran
Ankit Bhaskar
Ankit Pruthi
Ankita Ratha
Ankita Satija
Ankur Puri
Ankur Warikoo
Annie Mathew
Annie Parker
Antara Choudhury
Antara Raychaudhury
Antonet Fernando
Anu Singh
Anubhav Bhatt
Anuja Dasgupta
Anupriya
Anurama Suresh
Anurup Gulabani
Anusan Hazo
Anushka Siddiqui

Anwesha Basu

Apekshit Khare

Apoorva Kamat

Apuroop Kypuram

Archana Mantri

Archana Murthy

Archana Sahal

Arjun Bhatia

Arjun Murthy

Arpitha Rao

Arun Gopalakrishnan

Aruna Balamurugan

Aruna Gopakumar

Aruna VN

Arushi Agrawal

Aseem Shrivastava

Ashish Tiwari

Ashish Naik

Ashley Bartowitz

Ashley Havera

Ashley Kuriakose

Ashley Ritchie

Ashmita Padia

Ashna Shah

Ashrith Deshpande

Ashwin Manghat

Ashwini Rao Holla

Ashwini Pai

Asmita Paul

Astha Gupta

Aveejeet Palit

Avni Ahuja

Ayaan Bansal

Ayan Chakraborty

Ayush Garg

Ayush Kumar

Aziz Koleilat

Azmeera Mannu

Baljinder Kaur

Beena Thomas

Beng Sim Ho

Bhadauria Sonam

Bhagwan Kendre

Bhanuvilas Bandale

Bharti Daswani

Bhaskar Narannagari

Bhavna Lakhwani

Bhoomika Parti

Bhumika Matlani

Bhushika Kapoor

Binodan Sarma

Brandon McGrath

Brindha Vijendran

Carolyn Cherrett

Cecilia Chung

Chainani Dhiraj G

Chainani Prashant

Chandni Singh

Chandrashekhar Wadekar

Chandrima Chatterjee

Charanyan Gopal

Chinmay Deshpande

Chitra Balasundar

Christopher Gillette

Daksh Pratap Singh

Dale Smiley

Danielle Lesch

Darpan Jain

Darshan Kurup

Debanshu Roy

Debayan Ghosh

Deeksha Bhat

Deepa Balakrishnan

Deepa Chacko

Deepak Bansal

Deepambika TJ

Deepika Chouhan

Deepika Anu

Deepika Chhillar

Deepika Ghosh

Deepika Sodhi

Deepita Shukla

Deepshikha Bhardwaj

Deepti Mohankumar

Dhanashree Prabhu

Dhritiman Bhuyan

Dhruv Sharma

Dikshita Dikshita

Dilip Wadhwani

Dimple Bangalore

Dimple Ramchandani

Dipasha Mukherji

Divya Divakaran

Divya Loganathan

Divyajot Singh

Divyan Kurup

Divyanshi Galla

Divyanshu Dhingra

Dolly Lal

Dr Varsha Nikam

Dr Vinodkumar Ukarde

Dr Gautomi Dutta

Dr Govind Kasle

Dr Nagraj Deshpande

Dr Nuttha Ungnapatanin

Dr Pratibha Deshpande

Dr Suthida Suvanvecho

Dr Veena Gupta

Dr Vidya Deshpande

Dr Rekha Deshpande

Drishti Mulani

Durga Mithra

Ekta Rathod

Elizabeth Bocarro

Esha Shah
Eshaa Daryanani
Eshita Baijal
Falgun Barot
Fauzia Naqvi
Feroza Engineer
Flynn Francisco
Francis Harry Roy S
Gabriela Carolus
Garemsa Brahma
Garima Arora
Garima Shewkani
Garima Shewkani
Garima Verma
Gaurav G
Gaurav Alugh
Gaurav Patel
Gaurav Sharma
Gautam Annojjula
Gautam Desai
Gayathri Sreedharan
Geeta Kadayaprath
Geetha Anand
Gunasekaran
    Sevugapperumal
Gurpreet Kaur
Hadley Bowling
Hammad Abedin
Hardeep Kaur
Hargopal Chawla
Hariharan Bojan
Harika Bukkapattanam
Harikishan Baswaraj
Haritha Alankrita
Harleen Kaur
Harnidh Kaur
Harsh Kansagra
Harsh Lohit

Hima Bista
Hoori Murjani
Hriniya Bose
Hrishikesh Joshi
Iain Rodger
Indu Anand
Indu Raja
Isha Nirola
Ishina Sakhrani
Ivy Nazareth
Iyer Anesh
Jack Widders
Jahanara Raza
James Botha
Jamie Jewell
Janaki Surendranath
Japnam Kair Bindra
Jawhar Mordani
Jayaraman Vijayaraghavan
Jayesh Shanbhag
Jeel Gandhi
Jesdee Charoenpanichsiri
Jessica Iacobucci
Jessica Waddell
Jisha Thomas
Jitesh Luthra
Joe Baby Joseph
John Mascarenhas
Jommy Thomas
Jordan Moskal
Joseph Lucas
Joshey John
Jyothi Atre
Jyothi Upadhya
Kamdar Punita
Kami Richmond
Kamlesh Verma
Kanika Agarwal

Kanta Samtani
Kanupriya Durve
Kapil Kumar Yanamandra
    Venkata
Karan Mordani
Karan Narang
Kareena Samtani
Karishma Chainani
Karthik Balakrishnan
Karthik Sukumaran
Kartika Menon
Karuna Pochampalli
Kashish Vyas
Kathleen Guinn
Kathy Gabriel
Kato Minori
Kaustubha Parkar
Keren Rambow
Khatija Aslam
Kiran Narwani
Koena Lahiri
Krishna Murthy
Krishna Prasad
Kshiti Gala
Kuheli Dey
Kumar Animesh
Kumara Swamy Ganji
Kumud Nandwani
Kunal Chowdhury
Kunal Sajnani
Kundhavi P
Lakshmi Himabindu
    Jonnalagadda
Lakshmi Mandavilli
Lakshmidevi Dhandapani
Latha Ganesan
Laxman Rao Deshpande
Li Ning Low

Lucia Casagranda
Madan Ganesh
    Velayudham
Madhumita Das
Madhurantika Sunil
Mahesh Primalani
Mahima Randhawa
Mahima Garg
Mahima Randhawa
Mahima Taneja
Malvika Chandiramani
Mamta Batra
Manali Bhagwat
Manbir Chyle
Maneesha Aluru
Manish Mahajan
Manish Mishra
Manish Rana
Manisha Koppala
Manita Sehgal
Manna Sankar
Mannan Amroliwala
Manoj Sajnani
Mario da Penha
Mariya Illyasova
Max York
Mayank Dhiman
Mayank Dixit
Mayuri Kane
Meenakshi Sharma Pathak
Meenu Sharma
Meera Ravi
Megha Raiyani
Megha Wadhwa
Meghana Koppala
Meghna Jaruhar
Meher Roy Chowdhury
Mehul Mandewalkar

Messiah Chatterjee
Michael Bergan
Michael Giansiracusa
Minal Shamdasani
Minde Kaur
Mini Vatsala
Mira Levin
Mohd Zakir Hussain
Mohini B
Monica Hariharan
Morgan Schroth
Mriganki Nagpal
Mrinal Singh
Mrinal Manvi
Mrinmayee Shelgikar
Mrs Meenakshi
    Muthuveerappan
Mukti Shah
Murali Balakrishnan
Nachiket Katti
Nadia Eesa
Nadine Bharwani
Nakul Gupta
Nandini Dubey
Nanyeli hernandez
Naresh Chandiramani
Naresh Kasula
Natasha Ramchandani
Natasha Sabnani
Natasha Zarine
Nathan Hoening
Navleen Kaur
Neelima Bandi
Neeraj Goel
Neety Rai .
Neha Mathews
Neha Sureka
Neil Borate

Neyna Bhushan
Nicholas Cheremeteff
Niharika Mittal
Niketh Sabbineni
Nikhil J
Nikhil Jois
Nikhil Kishore
Nikhila Kanakamedala
Nikhilesh Ponde
Nikhitha Murali
Nikita Bandale
Nikita Gurudath
Nikita Kamdar
Nikita Mittal
Nilesh Pritam
Nina Bijoor
Nirav Shah
Nirmal Paul
Nirmal Murmu
Nirmallya Kar
Nisha Ramchandani
Nisha Shah
Nisha Verma
Nishant Dsouza
Nishant Singh
Niti Joshi
Nitin Bahuguna
Nitin Gandhi
Nitin Toopran
Nitin Tople
Nitya Mandewalker
Noby Thomas Cyriac
Ojas Gupta
Padma Rudraraju
Padmaja Chauhan
Palki Bhattacharyya
Pallabi Roy
Pankaj Kohli

Parima Panpruet

Parminder Gulati

Parth Asnani

Parv Sharma

Pavan Kumar Pillalamarri

Pavarit Chandhaprayoon

Paveena K

Pavithra RV

Pawan Reddy Ulindala

Philippa Walker

Piti Patcharavalai

Piuli Roy Chowdhury

Pooja Chandna

Pooja Dewoolkar

Pooja Sikund

Poonam Ponde

Poorva Joshi

Pragya Baweja

Pragya Purang

Prajwol Nepal

Prakash Chandiramani

Prakash Kamdar

Prakash Lalwani

Pramada Tirumala

Pramath Sinha

Pramod Cavale

Pranav Mehta

Pranav Singhal

Pranoy Sarkar

Prasanna Kumar

Prasenjit Chaudhuri

Prashant Gautam

Prashanth Balakrishnan

Prashanthi Y

Prashasti Singh

Prashenjit Pal

Prasiddha Rama Rao

Prateek Panchratana

Prathima Arun

Pratibha Devbhankar

Pratibha Rai

Pratik Deshpande

Preethi Bhaskaran

Preethi Premkumar

Preeti Singh

Preeti Golani

Prekshya Maharana

Prerna Khemani

Prima Virani

Prithi Radhakrishnan

Prithvi Arun

Priti Raje

Priya Baruah

Priya Dhanapal

Priya Narwani

Priya Srini

Priyakshi Saikia

Priyanka Krishna

Priyanka Prabhakar

Prof. Chayya Katti

PT J

Pujasree Konwar

Pushkar Lele

R Mathangi Chandramouli

Rachana Ramchand

Rachel Stevens

Rachit Monga

Radhika Piplani

Radhika Ralhan

Rag Ranjan

Ragini Thakur

Rahel Wohlhage

Rahila Rashid

Rahul Daswani

Rahul Mandewalker

Rahul Thadani

Rajat Nayyar

Rajeev Lochan Seth

Rajendra Paknikar

Rajendra Ponde

Rajesh Hathiramani

Rakesh Samtani

Rakhi Khialani

Raksha Sajnani

Rakshit Suri

Ralf Theune

Rama Krishna Janamanchi

Rama Vedachalam

Ramamurti Balasubramaniam

Ramarao Sayarwar

Ramchand Divya

Ramchander Namani

Ramesh Chennagiri

Ranjitha Janardhan

Rashi Daswani

Rashmeet Taluja

Ravi Singh

Rebecca Johnson

Rekha Prashanth

Rekha Garg

Reshma Varghese

Rimjhim Roy

Rimmy Khurana

Rishiraj Sinha

Rita Khurana

Ritika Arora

Ritu Arora

Rohan Banja

Rohan Nandi

Rohini Singh

Rohit Kumar

Rohit Manikandan

Rohit Rolla

Romina Kripalani

Ronit Sarkar

Ronojoy Bhuyan

Roopa Rajesh

RS Janwadkar

Ruchika Tulshyan

Rukmini Giridhar

Rukmini Das

Rukumini Bai Deshpande

Rupani Karishma

Rupani Sneha

Ryan Barrett

S Chandrasekhar

S Gopalakrishnan

S Prabhakar

Sachin Dev

Sachin Ghanwar

Sachin Paranjape

Sachin Serigar

Saee Tendulkar

Sai Naware

Sai Kumar

Sairoshini Daswani

Sajitha Narayanan

Sakshi Patil

Samar Pratap Singh

Samarjit Sinha

Sambandam Anand

Samit Bhandari

Sandeep Mehta

Sandeep Onkar

Sandhya Daswani

Sandhya Taklikar

Sangeeta Jagadesh

Sangeeta Sengupta

Sanila Samuel

Sanjay Buradkar

Sanjay Das

Sanjay Moorjani

Sanjna Malpani

Santosh Poluri

Santosh Sundaresan

Santosh Abraham

Sarita Santoshini

Saritha S

Sarmishta Mani

Sasidharan Kokkath

Sasiprabha Ramaswamy

Sathiya Priya
Ranganathan

Satyam Kumar Rai

Saumita Banerjee

Saumya Seth

Saurabh Sharma

Schitij Kulshrestha

Sean Kim

Sean Pinto

Seema Chowdhry

Seema Puthyapurayil

Senthilkumar Rajendran

Serena Jaffer

Shaefali Verma

Shahid Rashid

Shaila Tanwani

Shakuntala Devulapally

Shalini Bagaria

Sham Krisha

Shamdasani Yogita

Shanthi Karunakaran

Sharad Shankar

Sharada Datar

Sharmila Lahiri

Sharmishtha Bhadra

Shashank Karmarkar

Shashank Dabriwal

Shashank Mehta

Shashiprabha Gupta

Sheena Golani

Shikha Jain

Shilpa Balagopalan

Shilpi Banerjee

Shiny Leo

Shirin Talreja

Shirish Raut

Shiv Sharma

Shivangi Verma

Shivani Raturi

Shivani Suresh

Shivansh Monga

Shivshankar Menon

Shiwani Gurwara

Shobhit Gupta

Shraddha Deshpande

Shreedevi Narayanan

Shreya Mishra

Shreyas Anand

Shreyasi Singh

Shrijata Mukherjee

Shrimoyee Mukherjee

Shriya Sundaram

Shruthi M S

Shruti Patil

Shruti Kapoor

Shubhangi Upadhyay

Shubhayan Sengupta

Shweta Rao

Shyam Gupta

Shyamashree Rudra

Simran Kahlon

Simran Rana

Simranpreet Singh Oberoi

Smita Ahuja

Smruti Das

Sneha

Sneha Hatwar

Sneha Lalwani

Snehil Basoya

Snigdha Agarwal

Snigdha Malayanur

Sohinder Singh

Somya John

Sonal Rajiv
  Karamchandani

Sonali Shelke

Sonali Ghanwar

Sonali Gupta

Sonali Malaviya

Sonam Uttamchandani

Sonia Lalwani

Sophia Philips

Soujanya Deshpande

Soumya B

Sowjanya Aligala

Sreerupa Biswas

Sreesathy Rajakrishnan

Sri Ram Deepak
  Chivukula

Sriharsha Devulapalli

Srini Srinivasan

Sruthi Venkatramani

Steffi Olickal

Steve George

Sudarshan Vasudevan

Suhas Raje

Sujata Hati Baruah

Sukanya Honkote

Sukanya Remesh

Sumit Mishra

Suneet Malhotra

Sunil Bhosle

Sunil Sunkara

Sunny Adnani

Sunny Agarwal

Sunny Sandhu

Surbhi Gaur

Suriyaprakash C

Susan Daniel

Sushil Sehgal

Sushma Subhashchandra

Swapna Mehta

Swapna Velma

Swapnil Sharma

Swapnil Sharma

Swara Mehta

Swasti Pal

Swathi T P

Swati Sapna

Taab Arshad

Tamanna Mordani

Tanita Abraham

Tanmay Shah

Tanvi Khemani

Tanya Wadhwani

Tarana Thangamma

Tarika Seth

Tariq Hazarika

Ted Ingling

Tejshvi Jain

Thanisha Sehgal

Theertha Raj

Thillaikkarasi Velayutham

Tian Yuan

Tirthankar Khaund

Trilok Guntuka

Udita Makhija

Ujjaval Buch

Uma Iyer

Uma Paranjape

Unnati Sharma

Urmila Patil

Usha Gopalan

Utkarsh Amitabh

Utkarsh Gupta

Utkarsh Rai

Vaibhav Agarwal

Vaishali Shetty

Valli Arunachalam

Vandhana Parkavi
  Valaguru

Vani Verma

Vanisha Kishore

Vanita Motwani Mody

Varsha Bhagchandani

Varun Khanna

Varun Shyam

Varun Vashi Khemaney

Venkata Susanth
  Chadalavada

Venkataraghavan
  Srinivasan

Venkatesh Raje

Vibha Iyer

Vidhushri Singhal

Vidya Devanathan

Vijay Deshpande

Vijay Khurana

Vijayan Parthasarathy

Vijender Deshpande

Vijeta Marthi

Vikas B

Vikas Thakkar

Vikash Vaibhav

Vikram Rai

Vikrant

Viky Bohra

Vindhya Gooty Gooty

Vineet Abraham

Vineeta Yadav

Vinu Krishnaswamy
Vipul Shetty
Viraen Vaswani
Viresh Vaswani
Vishal Advani
Vishal Janani
Vishal Sajnani
Vishaya Tolani

Vishwas Sankhe
Vrinda Prahladka
Vrushali Ponde
Wadhwani Tina
Wadhwani Tushar
William Millhaem
Yashaswini Dayama
Yashna Lakhani

Yashodhara Lal
Yazmin Daryanani
Zahara Binti Latib
Zaini Baroom
Zarine Zarine
Zeina Chakhtoura

RICH MAN'S DISEASE

If you have tried to watch something on YouTube recently, you might be familiar with this—you click play and suddenly there's a video or a picture of a baby and there's someone crying and asking for help. If this sounds familiar, what you have encountered is a campaign video trying to raise funds for medical treatment. At this point, you may click "skip ad" or choose to donate. No judgements here. I belonged to the "skip ad" gang until the day I found myself having to think about starting a campaign to raise funds for my own treatment. If you have read the book this far, you know that it presents the experiences of cancer survivors and patients, so I won't spend too much time on setting the context of my illness, except to say that I had it and now had to potentially raise money to treat it. And raise lots of it. Like enough to buy a small apartment in Bengaluru and a fairly big one in Timbuktu.

If my real estate comparisons are not painting a clear picture, let me get into the numbers. At one point during my treatment, we were looking at having to raise up to thirty-five lakhs for a specialized treatment. I hope you're drinking a beverage at this point so you can spit it out for dramatic effect. Yes, specialized treatments for cancer are *that* expensive. In fact, I have also seen a treatment fundraiser with the target of over one crore. Turns out, fighting for your life is expensive. I know what you're thinking. That's why you should buy insurance, silly. I have insurance and it didn't help me. In the interests of being fair, I will start my story by talking about the time that insurance did help me.

I belong to the school of writing where every story must have an exotic setting. Mine is set in Finland in the year 2014 when I was an exchange student. My experience was postcard perfect except for a small wound, which, thanks to my foolhardiness, turned into a full-blown pus-filled abscess. Whoever received lemons from life has been really lucky, because it's mostly been brinjals in my basket. Predictably, my abscess decided to burst two days before I was scheduled to leave Finland. As I sat on a bus, leaking blood and pus, it still hadn't sunk in that I may have to seek medical attention. My Finnish friend, who was training to be a midwife at the time, dressed my wound as best as she could, and we decided to wait and watch. The next morning, my wound was still leaking so we decided to go to a clinic. The doctor took a look and referred me to a big hospital. The fact that my wound emitted an odor might give you an idea about how badly my wound was infected. I don't think everyday wounds are supposed to smell. So off to the hospital we went.

At the big hospital, I waited for the on-duty doctor to become available while the anesthesia kicked in. For a brief moment, the abscess became bearable. Next thing I knew, the doctor was prodding around my wound while I tried not to show any signs of weakness. In my mind, I was representing my country, and we are not a nation of weaklings. After all, I was a grown-up now. Once my wound was dressed, I was told I could leave. No hefty bill, thanks to socialism! *Kiitos paljon!* Thanks a lot!

Fast forward to a few months later—a hefty bill in Euros shows up at my house in Bengaluru. By this point, I had already returned to university to continue my studies. My dad called me, asking what the hell was happening. That's when I remembered I had bought insurance during the exchange trip. I had no idea whether they would accept it, but I filed a claim anyway. I can't stress enough how cumbersome it was. Zeus should have just made Sisyphus file an insurance claim for eternity. It's almost as if the process is the punishment for making them pay for your treatment. But as they say, all's well that ends well. The insurance company paid for my